AN ETHICAL FRAMEWORK FOR COMPLEMENTARY AND ALTERNATIVE THERAPISTS

Julie Stone

1954088

LIBRARY

ACC. No. 36061852.

DEPT.

CLASS No.

UNIVERSITY OF CHESTER

London and New York

First published 2002
by Routledge
11 New Fetter Lane, London EC4P 4EE

Simultaneously published in the USA and Canada
by Routledge
29 West 35th Street, New York, NY 10001

Routledge is an imprint of the Taylor & Francis Group

© 2002 Julie Stone

Typeset in Times by Taylor & Francis Books Ltd
Printed and bound in Great Britain by TJ International Ltd, Padstow, Cornwall

All rights reserved. No part of this book may be reprinted or
reproduced or utilised in any form or by any electronic,
mechanical, or other means, now known or hereafter
invented, including photocopying and recording, or in any
information storage or retrieval system, without permission in
writing from the publishers.

British Library Cataloguing in Publication Data
A catalogue record for this book is available from the British Library

Library of Congress Cataloging in Publication Data
Stone, Julie.
An ethical framework for complementary and alternative therapists / Julie Stone.
Includes bibliographical references and index.
1. Alternative medicine–Moral and ethical aspects. I. Title.

R733 .S865 2002
174'.2–dc21   2001058714

ISBN   0–415–27890–2 (hbk)
ISBN   0–415–27900–3 (pbk)

CONTENTS

v

CONTENTS

PREFACE

Complementary and alternative medicine, or CAM, is a boom industry. Whilst many cultures across the globe have always relied on traditional forms of healing, high levels of usage of alternative forms of health care are now evident in all developed nations. More people in the USA are now thought to consult CAM therapists than primary health physicians. What is particularly remarkable is that this transition has occurred mostly in the private sector, with individuals seeking out and often paying for these therapies themselves, notwithstanding free access to conventional medicine. Whereas in the past, non-conventional approaches to health could be dismissed by the medical establishment as a marginal activity, they are now part of mainstream culture and are seen and used by the public as a viable and accessible alternative to western allopathic medicine.

The growth of consumer interest in CAM therapies has prompted calls for greater integration with orthodox medicine, so that all patients may benefit from its perceived advantages. Although few health systems are truly pluralistic, many examples of integrated practice are beginning to emerge in the USA, the UK and elsewhere. However, despite the growing professionalisation of many therapies, and the greater attention given to training and establishing competencies, concerns remain about *standards* within CAM. These concerns are coming from the medical and nursing professions, from would-be purchasers and insurers, and from members of the public.

For some time, the primary medical objection to CAM therapies has centred around whether these therapies work. In determining this issue, little weight has been given to the subjective voices of patients who feel that they have benefited as a result of these treatments. Critics of CAM are dismissive of anecdotal reports of efficacy and calls have been made for scientific proof that these therapies work. This comes at a time when conventional medicine itself has had to face up to its own lack of evidence. As conventional medicine becomes ever more evidence-based, there has been increasing pressure to subject CAM therapies to the same level of scientific scrutiny. With the focus firmly fixed on effectiveness, the ethical implications raised by the

CAM therapeutic encounter have been paid little or no attention. To the extent that these issues have been considered at all, it has been presumed that the issues simply mirror those arising between doctors and patients. This goes hand in hand with a tacit assumption that CAM relationships do not give rise to many ethical issues because CAM therapists rarely deal with life and death situations.

This view could not be more misguided. All health care encounters give rise to ethical considerations. At the heart of the therapeutic encounter is a practitioner/patient relationship based on trust, need, dependency and hope. Patients expect to be consulted, to be heard and to be treated competently whenever they are consulting a health practitioner. These expectations give rise to ethical responsibilities quite distinct from the technical competencies required of any practitioner. Practitioners face moral dilemmas every day. Should they ever tell 'white lies' to spare their patients' feelings? How can they maintain a professional stance, yet not appear too remote? How much of themselves should they reveal to patients? What should they do when clients are obviously attracted to them? How long should they continue to treat patients whose self-harming behaviour is hindering therapeutic progress? How directive should they be in encouraging patients to leave a destructive relationship?

Within CAM relationships, the dynamics and parameters of the therapeutic relationship may pose additional ethical issues. Conventionally, a successful therapeutic outcome is the removal of symptoms or the management of a chronic condition. CAM therapies attempt to treat the underlying cause of a disease as well as the symptoms, in the hope that they will prevent ill health from arising in the future. As such, the measures to determine outcome may need to be broader than those used in conventional medicine. Patients consulting CAM therapists expect to take an active role in their own healing process and do not necessarily view the therapist as the technical expert with all the answers. Many clients do not view themselves as ill at all, but are turning to CAM to enhance their well-being. This, too, changes the nature of the ethical relationship between the parties.

These factors, together with the political, economic and cultural context within which these activities take place, call for a reappraisal of the ethics of the CAM therapeutic relationship. It is wrong to assume that tighter regulation obviates the need to discuss the ethics of CAM encounters. External regulation may offer general guidance to practitioners and curb the worst excesses of unprofessional behaviour, but ultimately, the responsibility to act ethically rests with the individual practitioner. The power of disciplinary boards to punish practitioners found guilty of professional misconduct may be one way of ensuring ethical conduct, but it has to be seen as part of a co-ordinated strategy of training and encouraging practitioners to be ethical. Since not all therapies meet current definitions of professions, or aspire to be considered as health professions, this book must look beyond the processes

employed by external regulatory bodies and consider theoretical and practical aspects of what it means for CAM practitioners to act ethically.

Consideration of the ethical dimensions of the therapeutic encounter is
timely for all therapists, irrespective of how their particular therapy is underpinned by evidence, or whether the therapy is currently licensed or regulated.
Practitioners can benefit or harm their patients whether or not the therapy is
supported by research or is regulated. Whilst offering a therapy that has not
been demonstrated to benefit a patient is a significant ethical issue in itself,
debate on the ethical implications of CAM cannot wait until political issues
such as integration and regulation are resolved.

CAM relationships, like all other health care relationships, require
consent, confidentiality, and the need to maintain safe boundaries. Although
CAM therapists may hold very different views about health and illness, the
substantive content of most healing encounters produces similar ethical
questions. This is not, of course, to suggest that all CAM therapies are the
same. The use of 'CAM' as an umbrella term to describe countless therapeutic approaches has historically been a device to denote the
marginalisation of CAM from conventional medicine. CAM therapies are
not a homogenous group. Clearly, CAM therapies are very different from
each other and different to allopathic medicine. But in terms of ethics, there
is greater similarity between health professionals than difference.

This book demonstrates that the ethical requirements of CAM practitioners are no less relevant than the ethics of any other group of health
professionals. The difference is one of emphasis and interpretation. To give
an example, the content and style of explaining risks to a patient and
gaining permission to treat may be very different for a hypnotherapist, a
chiropractor or a surgeon, but the underlying rationale of respecting the
patient's autonomy is the same for all three and needs to be understood by
each group of practitioners.

Whilst recognising the large degree of commonality between all health
professionals, the alternative basis of CAM practice raises fundamental
epistemological questions about the nature of ethics. If the philosophies
underpinning CAM are at odds with the dominant theories of disease
causation and disease management, can we assume that these are merely
technical differences which have no bearing on the philosophical question of
how CAM practitioners ought to behave? Much of the literature in bioethics
views the doctor/patient relationship as the paradigmatic example of a
health care encounter. Various assumptions are made about the roles of
'good' doctors and 'good' patients, gender, dominant cultural values, patient
expectations and a shared (western) understanding of health and disease.
These assumptions may not be shared by many CAM practitioners or,
indeed, CAM patients. Can the language and constructs of bioethics be
invoked in analysing CAM relationships? Bioethics is grounded in, and a
product of, the dominant biomedical paradigm. Western values and western

preoccupation with the rights of the individual underpin traditional discussions of what it means to be an ethical health practitioner. Is this an appropriate framework within which to judge the moral actions of CAM practitioners, whose therapies may be grounded in different philosophical traditions, with profoundly different cultural assumptions about the role of patients and healers?

This question has never been more relevant, and is prompted by the extent to which patients are demonstrating their enthusiasm for CAM by voting with their feet. Integration of CAM practitioners or CAM practices into conventional medicine is becoming a reality and the ethical probity of CAM practitioners will be an important factor in the integration debate. But it may be short sighted to assume that the ethical tools invoked in conventional medicine will provide an adequate or optimal basis for the conduct of CAM practitioners. Tension exists precisely because integration, at least at present, is taking the form of integration of CAM into mainstream medicine where certain beliefs and assumptions about ethics already exist. In much the same way as doctors expect CAM research to follow the gold standard of randomised control trials, there is an unspoken assumption that CAM practitioners can be more readily integrated into orthodox health care settings if they have similar codes of ethics and similar regulatory structures. This expectation is naïve because it overlooks the different relationship between medicine and the state and CAM therapies and the state. Whereas the former relationship is legitimised, with doctors, in certain situations, authorised to act as agents of the state, the very existence of CAM represents a challenge to the existing medico-political hegemony.

This book probes the differences between CAM and other therapeutic approaches to see if there are genuine ethical differences in how the relationship might be construed which might require different forms of governance. Comparisons will be drawn with conventional medicine, not because the doctor/patient relationship represents an ideal standard of care, but because modern medicine represents the dominant discourse of health and healing. This impacts on every aspect of the therapeutic encounter, from how healing relationships are regulated, how patients' expectations of healing encounters are shaped, and how CAM is inevitably constructed as 'other'.

Professional codes of ethics also have a legalistic basis, so that the recommendations for ethical practice are a synthesis of ethical and legal requirements. All health care practitioners, including CAM therapists, must work within the laws of the country in which they are practising, and if the law of the land requires practitioners to obtain consent or respect patient confidentiality, this applies no less to CAM practitioners than to any other health care practitioner.

The purpose of this book is primarily two-fold. At a theoretical level, it will attempt to question what is meant by ethics. Do different people share a common morality, which can shed light on how practitioners ought to behave, or does each culture or community have its own set of morals which reflect the values and needs of that particular society? This inquiry will hopefully shed light on whether it is justifiable to apply traditional bioethical ethical theories to analyse the CAM relationship. If it emerges that the western, consumerist model is not relevant to therapies grounded in different philosophical traditions, it may be necessary to construct an alternative basis for analysing the ethical implications of CAM therapeutic encounters. Secondly, this book is intended as a practical guide for CAM therapists, CAM students and CAM patients. Using case studies from CAM practice, major ethical topics will be discussed. These will identify key ethical dilemmas which practitioners are most likely to encounter in the course of professional practice, and suggest practical solutions to enhance the therapeutic relationship to the benefit of patient and practitioner.

Accordingly, Part I demonstrates that all health care relationships give rise to ethical, as well as legal and professional, responsibilities. Since external regulatory controls, including legal and disciplinary proceedings, operate retrospectively, they only come into play when a patient has already been harmed. This book focusses on what it means for practitioners to act ethically and is intended to make therapists reflect critically on their own practice, to prevent harm from arising, and to learn how to resolve ethical tensions as and when they do present. This part of the book will draw on and discuss three sources of ethical guidance currently available to practitioners, namely: existing bioethical theories, professional codes of ethics, and the parts of the law which affect professional practice. Suggestions will be offered as to how these may need to be developed to respond to the nuances of CAM practice.

Part II concentrates on the commonality between health professionals and considers the major ethical issues raised by therapeutic practice, including competence to practise, consent, confidentiality and maintaining boundaries. These key issues are not therapy-specific. Rather, they are central to all CAM health care relationships. Examples will be given from a wide range of therapies to demonstrate how ethical principles might need to be interpreted in different situations.

In Part III, groups of therapies will be considered on the basis of the unique ethical issues they raise. This novel classification will find some unlikely therapies being discussed side by side, and is intended to stimulate thought on the ethical aspects of therapies rather than their therapeutic approach. Acupuncture, colonic irrigation and chelation therapy may not seem to have much in common when one applies traditional classifications, but they share the commonality of being highly invasive procedures which carry inherent risks. From an ethical point of view, avoidance of harm and obtaining consent will be highly relevant. Similarly, product-based therapies, such as homoeopathy, herbalism and Ayurveda, share other distinct ethical issues around quality control, patient expectations about prescribing and the acceptability of using placebos. Quite different issues are raised by hands-on therapies, in which boundary issues, consent and the ethics of treating vulnerable groups dominate.

It is hoped that this book will be useful for practitioners and students of CAM, for conventional health care practitioners with an interest in CAM, for patients using CAM, and for policy-makers influencing decisions about the integration of complementary and alternative therapies and mainstream medicine. Whilst professional bodies have an important role in developing these debates, ultimately, whether a practitioner acts ethically is down to the individual. In providing tools for critical, reflective practice, it is hoped that the CAM therapeutic relationship can be strengthened; the capacity for healing will then be enhanced and innovative practice will flourish.

1

INTRODUCTION

Given the growth in the last twenty years of the professional literature on bioethics, readers might legitimately ask whether it is necessary to devote an entire book to the ethics of complementary and alternative medicine (CAM). After all, the side effects and risks of complementary medicine are generally perceived to be lower than in conventional medicine. So many people now consult CAM practitioners that this would suggest high levels of patient satisfaction. To the extent that ethical issues arise, are these any different to the issues arising in other health care relationships? Could an ethically curious therapist not simply extract the necessary information from a conventional health care ethics text, substituting the words 'complementary therapist' for 'doctor' or 'nurse'?

Given the growing awareness of ethical responsibilities amongst other health care professions, a strong argument needs to be made as to why CAM therapists should be treated differently from other health care professionals as far as ethical responsibilities are concerned. Arguably, the more that CAM practitioners organise themselves professionally like orthodox practitioners, and the greater the level of integration within orthodox health care systems, the closer any model of ethics for CAM practitioners should resemble that which pertains to other health professionals. If we accept the basic premise that patients consult health professionals with a desire to be healed, and that all health carers, in whatever way, seek to benefit patients, should there not be a single ethical framework which applies to all health care practitioners, be they spiritual healers or surgeons?

At first sight, this seems to be an attractive proposition. If one takes the example of sexual abuse of a patient by a practitioner, it ought to make little difference in regulatory terms whether the abusing practitioner is a physiotherapist or an acupuncturist. Creating and maintaining safe boundaries is critical whatever the therapeutic orientation of the practitioner. Similarly, a patient needs to be informed of the risk of serious injury from neck manipulation no less than the risks of spinal surgery since in each case, the information will be vital to the patient's ability to make an informed choice as to whether to proceed with the treatment. Yet, despite the seeming similarity, CAM practice raises profound and novel questions for ethicists. The very features which differentiate CAM therapeutic encounters from relationships with conventional health care practitioners create unique ethical dilemmas. An ethical investigation of the CAM therapeutic encounter needs to ask the following:

- Should the normal risk/benefit analysis be applied to the last resort patient who has exhausted every available conventional form of medication, and now wishes to seek complementary approaches, however outlandish and untested? Should parents be entitled to make that decision if their child is dying and the parents have lost confidence in conventional medicine?
- What complaints mechanism can realistically compensate a patient who has paid $100 to have their aura cleansed but feels no different at the end of the session than at the start? Should we give people the freedom to spend their money as they wish or protect potentially vulnerable patients from exploitation?
- What ethical principles should apply when the client is not 'ill' as conventionally defined, and views the therapeutic encounter as an opportunity to enhance their well-being? If the therapeutic encounter is reconceptualised as being about health improvement or enhancement as well as treating ill health, should the same ethical principles apply? If a patient views their weekly aromatherapy massage or reflexology session on a par with a visit to the hairdresser or manicurist, should the former be subject to a more restrictive ethical framework and if so, why?
- How can therapeutic outcomes be measured or compared to conventional medicine when a central goal of CAM therapy is to prevent the patient from getting ill?
- Can the 'competencies' of a psychic healer, for example, be discussed within the same discourse as a discussion of the competencies of a surgeon?
- If successful therapeutic outcomes depend, in part, on active patient involvement and patient self-responsibility, does this mean that patients must agree to become informed about what the therapist is doing to them, and participate in shared decision-making? Can CAM therapists work with patients who refuse to help themselves and prefer to be a passive recipient of treatment given by the therapist?
- If self-responsibility is essential to the healing process, does that mean that different ethical principles should apply in relation to the treatment of children and mentally incapacitated patients who are unlikely to be able to bring about the substantial lifestyle changes recommended by therapists?

These examples demonstrate that the content and context of the CAM therapeutic encounter may require a very different ethical analysis. An important preliminary point is that not all aspects of the therapeutic encounter are morally controversial. Ethicists tend to focus on worst-case scenarios and may even go looking for dilemmas where none exist. Indeed, formalised study of bioethics may falsely lead one to think that there is a 'right thing to do' in any given situation.[1] Many practitioners, when asked, say that they have never encountered an ethical dilemma in practice. Perhaps a generous interpretation of such a claim is that 'good' practitioners instinctively act ethically and resolve tensions before they escalate. It is not the purpose of this book to go looking for problems where none exist. A probable reason why very few people sue or complain about CAM practitioners is that therapists are genuinely more in tune with their patients. Hopefully most CAM practitioners do practise ethically. The levels of high patient satisfaction with CAM would surely bear this out.

Nonetheless, it is equally possible that practitioners who claim they have never encountered an ethical dilemma have an insufficiently developed awareness as to what constitutes an ethical issue. Gut instincts may currently guide practitioners through the complexities of therapeutic relationships, but these are not an adequate substitute for rigorous, reflective analysis of the ethical basis of the therapeutic encounter. CAM relationships do clearly give rise to a range of ethical issues, and hopefully all practitioners, however experienced, will find useful tools in this book to help them to refine their moral sensibilities and to reflect on how better to resolve ethical dilemmas which may arise in the future. Patients also have to exercise self-responsibility, since they too share some of the moral responsibility within the therapeutic exchange, an issue often overlooked in duty-based bioethics which concentrates on the practitioner's duties towards the patient. Deciding what is ethically appropriate cannot be divorced from the principles and values that underpin practice and the needs and expectations of clients. These will now be explored.

Are there shared CAM values and characteristics?

A useful starting point for analysis is to ascertain whether there are any shared values which underpin CAM practice. To the extent that CAM comprises nearly two hundred different therapeutic modalities, are there any common themes that characterise the practice of complementary and alternative medicine which will influence the ethical implications of these sorts of therapeutic encounters? Is it possible to find statements which cover all therapists when the range of complementary and alternative therapies is so diverse, ranging from whole systems (such as Traditional Chinese Medicine, Ayurveda and homoeopathy and herbalism), to diagnostic methods (such as iridology and kinesiology), and self-help methods (such as yoga and biofeedback)?

The Chantilly Report[2], produced as a result of a US workshop involving more than two hundred experts on CAM, divided therapies into seven broad categories of holistic practice, namely: (1) mind/body interventions; (2)

bioelectromagnetics applications in medicine; (3) alternative systems of medical practice; (4) manual healing methods; (5) pharmacological and biological treatments not yet accepted by mainstream medicine; (6) herbal medicine; and (7) treatments focussing on diet and nutrition in the prevention and treatment of chronic disease. This gives some idea of the diversity of interventions under discussion. The question is whether these different categories share common values or approaches to health and healing which may better direct our inquiry of the ethical issues which their practice might raise.

Until recently, the only common link between CAM therapies was their absence from the orthodox medical school curriculum and the unwillingness of health insurers to reimburse patients for using these therapies. Indeed, the Harvard definition of alternative medicine *is* one of exclusion from mainstream medicine. Recent studies, however, demonstrate that this definition of exclusion can no longer be relied upon. As Eisenberg *et al.*'s 1997 follow-up study reveals, an increasing number of US insurers and managed care organisations now offer alternative medicine programmes and benefits[3], and the majority of US medical schools and health care institutions elsewhere now offer courses on alternative medicine.[4]

For our current purpose, Eskinazi offers a more fruitful definition of alternative medicine:

> I propose that alternative medicine be defined as a broad set of health care practices (ie, already available to the public) that are not readily integrated into the dominant health care model, because they pose challenges to diverse societal beliefs and practices (cultural, economic, scientific, medical, and educational). This definition brings into focus factors that may play a major role in the a priori acceptance or rejection of various alternative health care practices by any society. Unlike criteria of current definitions, those of the proposed definition would not be expected to change significantly without significant societal changes.[5]

This is a useful definition because it demonstrates the full extent to which CAM poses a threat to prevailing orthodoxies. In highlighting the various challenges alternative medicine poses, Eskinazi clarifies the point that acceptance or rejection by the medical profession is no longer the main or sole issue, because alternative medicine challenges a far broader range of beliefs. For this reason, integration of CAM and conventional medicine will never be a matter of mere therapeutics.

Given that there is rarely consensus even amongst members of the same therapy, is it realistic to hope to find values which cut across CAM as a whole? In order to make a meaningful transition from collective values to collective ethical precepts, we should not be lured into uncritical reliance upon some of the values therapists claim to possess. For example, we ought not to accept uncritically the contention that all complementary therapists work holistically, or that all therapists are patient-centred in their approach, without trying to establish what this might mean to individual practitioners and, perhaps more importantly, what patients think these terms mean.

The following is a possible list of shared values which might underpin the CAM therapeutic encounter. These values may apply to some therapies and therapists more than others and need to be discussed in turn. Perhaps no practitioner would identify with all of the following characteristics, but each raises issues that impact on the ethical relationship between practitioners and patients.

The holistic view of patients and of illness

The vast majority of CAM practitioners use the term 'holistic' to describe their practice. The most common use of the term holism refers to treating the patient as a whole person. Thus, illness is not just a physical phenomenon, but an indication of an imbalance which may relate to the patient's mind, body and spirit. Because of this, many practitioners might start by working on physical symptoms, but would also seek to find and treat the underlying problem. The holistic approach is starkly at odds with the reductionist biomedical model which views the ill patient in similar terms to faulty machinery and seeks to remove physical symptoms rather than treating underlying causes. If the concern is with the whole person, then it becomes more realistic for a single practitioner to treat a patient, rather than the system of specialisation within orthodox medicine, where a patient may be referred to several specialists who only treat bits of the person. As Sharma asks:

> If the patient is a whole person, then does it make sense to have completely different teams of people dealing with his/her musculo-skeletal system, digestive tract, mental health etc.?[6]

Interrelated aspects of holism are that the whole amounts to more than the sum of its parts and that individual health cannot be seen in isolation, but as part of society and the environment. Although the notion of holism has extended beyond the practice of alternative therapies, Douglas asserts that true holism is 'a philosophy of the body which does not grow out of the history of western medicine'. She maintains that there is a distinct difference between what a complementary practitioner means by working holistically and what a western-trained physician who claims to work holistically means. She describes the difference thus:

> Our doctor's holism stops at the boundaries of the body and stays within the boundaries of the medical profession, whereas holistic

medicine takes global account of the patient's whole personality and spiritual environment.[7]

The holistic dimensions of the CAM relationship may raise ethical issues not present in a relationship which takes a more mechanistic view of patients and their illness. One concern is the tendency of practitioners to give advice on their patient's lifestyle and emotional well-being, even if they have not been specifically trained to do so.

> *A recently qualified herbalist is treating a woman for depression. Over the course of several sessions, it emerges that his patient feels trapped within her arranged marriage, and is a victim of psychological and physical abuse. The herbalist, who is trying to be supportive, encourages his patient to leave her husband, and provides her with information about refuges. She is grateful for his help and leaves home. Subsequently, he is horrified to read in the local paper that his patient has been tracked down by her husband and savagely attacked. The herbalist receives a threatening phone call telling him to mind his own business or face the consequences.*

This example shows what can happen when practitioners impose their personal values on their patients, in this case his belief that women have a right to be free from a violent husband. Although the therapist is not directly responsible for the attack, this case illustrates the dangers of offering directive advice, without the training to do so, and without taking into account cross-cultural difficulties, specifically about women's right to autonomy, a value prized in the west, but interpreted differently in more traditional cultures.

Ideally, a holistic relationship will be one in which the views of the individual are given considerable prominence, as the patient's emotional and spiritual issues are less readily measurable by external forms of observation and rely on the patient communicating his/her subjective experience to the practitioner. Where practitioners work in co-operation with patients, there will hopefully be less scope for the practitioner to tell the patient what to do, and more opportunity for active listening on the part of the practitioner and negotiating an appropriate course of action.

Holistic practice is not unique to complementary and alternative medicine. Many conventional physicians would like to work more holistically, but their attempts to do so are often constrained by time pressures. A practitioner who elicits information and directs a cure relating to the patient's physical, emotional and spiritual state is likely to spend a long time with the patient. The time spent on the consultation is likely to be beneficial in itself and is identified by Cohen as one of the main reasons that patients do not sue complementary therapists even if something goes wrong.[8]

Many eastern therapies see humans and their natural surroundings as inseparable, with health or imbalance in the environment affecting the health of individuals. Yet most western ethical theories consider only how people ought to behave towards other people and pay little or no attention to people's moral duties towards other species, or towards the environment. As an ethical issue, how much energy should CAM practitioners devote to lobbying on environmental issues which will impact on the health of their individual patients and society in general? Whilst orthodox doctors have shied away from such areas as being outside the realm of medicine, holistic practice might require a more political stance as an aspect of patient advocacy.

An ethical concern borne out of the holistic model of treatment relates to the increased potential for harm when health carers claim to treat emotional and spiritual health. A practitioner who hopes to be able to bring about changes in a patient's physical, emotional and spiritual state might also be capable of causing harm in these spheres. This issue is particularly explicit in some indigenous healing practices, which can be used to bring about harm as well as benefit. Far from suggesting that CAM practitioners would deliberately intend to cause harm or distress to their patients, the point needs to be made that healing endeavours which can have a therapeutic effect may also cause a patient harm.

Whereas one tends to think of harm from unsuccessful therapy as meaning physical harm, practitioners who explicitly work with patients' emotions may, however unintentionally, cause that person psychological harm. This is most likely to occur if the practitioner fails to recognise that the client is severely, emotionally damaged or suffering from a psychiatric disorder, or where the CAM practitioner is insufficiently equipped to manage the consequences of stirring up emotional issues. Whilst newly qualified practitioners have greater familiarity with western medical concepts, they may be less able to spot a patient who is seriously psychotic rather than mildly neurotic. This highlights the need for rigorous training if, in practice, the emotional component of working holistically is akin to providing counselling or psychotherapy. To call oneself a holistic practitioner is to imply that one has the competence to meet the physical, emotional and spiritual needs of a patient. This competence is unlikely to be acquired in a training lasting only a few weeks or months.

Many holistic practitioners would reject this legalistic breakdown of holistic practice into distinct physical, emotional and spiritual competencies. They would argue that such an analysis rests upon the assumption that there is a mind/body split (sometimes referred to as Cartesian thinking or mind/body dualism). Practitioners would assert that physical, emotional and spiritual health cannot be neatly divided into three as though they were separate, unrelated entities. As Fulder explains:

> Oriental medicine and the major alternative medical systems never passed a Cartesian phase, so there is no need to postulate or evoke concepts like psychosomatic, or even autonomy. These are qualities observed naturally within the mind–body–heart continuum, expressed as the total energetic body of man.[9]

This argument may have validity for ancient healing traditions but is less applicable to many 'New Age' therapies. Fulder's point, does, however, have profound ramifications for any analysis of ethics of the CAM therapeutic relationship. It denotes how very different the paradigmatic basis of CAM therapies are from the biomedical model. The implications for ethical theory are very significant because western bioethics places individual autonomy at the centre of ethical analysis, and presumes that moral action involves rational moral agents.

Although CAM practitioners may reject this model in terms of how they treat, they need to be aware that, in terms of how CAM therapies are governed, western models of regulation are bound by the same dualistic, material assumptions which underscore the biomedical model. Ethical and legal rules do attempt to respect the patient's autonomy and do distinguish between physical harm and emotional harm. If a practitioner is sued, lawyers will try to establish cause and effect even if CAM therapists do not think there is a linear relationship between the treatment given and the patient's response.

Focus on the uniqueness of the individual

Rather than matching the patient's symptoms to a disease process and offering standardised therapy for that condition, CAM therapists tend to diagnose on the totality of issues presented by the individual patient. Each patient is different and has a unique constitution, requiring individualised treatment. Conventional medicine, in contrast, treats patients on the basis of objective symptoms, with treatments which are tailored towards the illness and not the individual. When new drugs are developed, they are designed to work on patient populations suffering from the same condition, on the basis that the similarities between patients are greater than their differences. This, argues Kottow, is one of medicine's downfalls:

> The main stumbling-block of a scientific approach has been that science operates with generalities whereas medicine has to act on sick individuals.... As science progresses, the individual *qua* individual appears to be side tracked from its benefits. It is hardly surprising that patients feel neglected by high-tech medicine and turn towards alternative approaches.[10]

Individual characteristics are only of clinical interest to conventional doctors in the case of inherited conditions and even then, treatment is not yet individualised in any real sense. Although work being carried out in human genetics is paving the way for individualised treatments which will take account of a patient's unique genetic make up, orthodox medicine looks for commonality, not individuality. Seen most starkly in the context of medical research, there is a failure to take account of the subject's race, culture, gender and socio-economic position, all of which are known to impact on health, but which are discounted when designing new drugs and treatments. CAM operates from the opposite starting point; that it is impossible to treat a patient *without* looking at his or her specific and unique circumstances. This is sometimes described as representing a 'patient-centred approach'. This is well summarised by Fulder:

> One of the indications of the richness of the medical system is the development of a typology in which individual differences in health, disease and response to the environment can be understood. For example, the constitutional picture in Ayurvedic medicine is a highly detailed art that integrates thousands of characteristics of body, skin, personality, habits, etc., defined in terms of Vata ('airiness'), Pitta ('fieriness') and Kapha ('wateriness'). This establishes an individual's susceptibilities, strengths, and weaknesses, and guides both prevention and treatment. By contrast, Western herbalism does not make extensive use of constitutional differences, and modern medicine ignores it completely unless there are inherited pathologies.[11]

The most obvious ethical implication is that patients are likely to derive optimal benefit from being treated as an individual. Each person experiences illness in a different way and the idea that a patient will really be heard and understood is extremely powerful. High levels of patient satisfaction suggest that patients respond well to an individualised approach. But treating the patient individualistically is not necessarily synonymous with respecting patients' autonomy, as many CAM practitioners would assert. Whilst commending the individualised approach in alternative medicine, Kottow asserts:

> Alternative approaches do concentrate on the individual, but they disparage the personal values by reducing the patient to the metaphysical and administrative order of their holistic perspective, where he becomes an acquiescing appendage.[12]

This statement questions the presumed value of CAM 'patient-centredness'. Critics of CAM argue that interest in the patient is not a substitute for effective treatment. Whilst patients do not generally like to have their autonomy overridden, most patients have sought out a health practitioner to be cured or made better in some respect. Lip service to respecting the patient's autonomy is of little value if the therapy offered is not beneficial.

The notion of individualised treatment also has implications for conducting research. Within biomedicine, the gold standard for clinical research is the randomised control trial (RCT). The purpose of an RCT is to test the effectiveness of a new drug or treatment in a carefully selected group of patients who, it is hoped, will benefit from the new treatment. A second group of patients (the control group) are given either best available therapy or a placebo (an inert substance, sometimes called a 'dummy pill') if there is no best effective treatment. The purpose of the control group is to see how the new treatment works in comparison to what is already available. The groups of patients are chosen according to very strict inclusion and exclusion criteria to make sure that treatment is being given to similar groups of patients. In a double blind trial, neither they, nor the doctor will know which treatment they are receiving, to reduce the possibility of bias.

The underlying theory is that if a therapy can be shown to demonstrate a particular effect in a given group, the results should be reproducible. If the treatment is successful in one group of patients with a particular symptom, it should be effective in other groups of patients with the same condition. The thinking behind RCTs, and indeed much of conventional medicine, is that the similarities between patients are greater than the differences, and that broadly speaking, a hundred patients suffering from the same symptoms can all be given the same treatment. So, for example, doctors might prescribe the same anti-histamine to 100 hayfever sufferers. CAM therapists, by contrast, view each patient as a unique individual. Accordingly, the manifestation of symptoms may have a profoundly different underlying cause from one patient to the next and may require quite different treatments. Similarly, the manifestation of a disease will present entirely differently from one patient to the next. Benefiting a patient may thus require a quite different approach from patient to patient. From a research perspective, the fact that a hundred different patients suffering from hayfever might each be given a *different* treatment makes it harder to systematically measure CAM efficacy.

Until relatively recently, such arguments have thwarted attempts to research CAM. Researchers in the past shied away from the challenge of devising methodologies to take account of this highly individualised way of working, or dismissed attempts to standardise individualised treatments for research purposes on the basis that this is not how the treatment would be delivered in practice. This position is no longer tenable. Clearly, a huge amount of empirical research into CAM has already been conducted. If patients, or groups of patients, or groups of symptoms, could never be compared, how did the original knowledge base for any given therapy develop in the first place? How did homoeopaths ever determine which remedies were good for which symptoms or acupuncturists learn which symptoms responded to which acupuncture points? Increasingly, it is accepted that CAM research can be carried out which takes account of the highly individualised nature of CAM practice and new approaches to CAM research methodology are evolving constantly. These issues will be taken up further in Part II.

Capacity for self-healing

Acknowledgement of the body's capacity to heal itself is a fundamental principle of most complementary and alternative therapies. The emphasis of many treatments is to restore a patient's vital force and promote the body's capacity to heal itself. Micozzi points out:

> If the body heals itself, has its own energy and is uniquely individual, then the focus is not on the healer but on the healed. Although this concept may be humbling to the practitioner as heroic healer, it is liberating to realize that in the end each person heals himself or herself. If the healer is not the sole source of health and healing, there is room for humility, as well as room for both patient and practitioner to participate in the interaction.[13]

CAM practitioners believe that the body, in the right environment, has great powers to heal itself and that often, what the therapist is doing is merely providing the tools for the body to heal itself and mobilising the body's natural self-healing response. Whilst the therapist may have technical expertise, the patient has an expertise of his or her own and the therapeutic relationship represents a genuine partnership or alliance between practitioner and patient. Lipson and Steiger note that:

> This holistic perspective continues to be present in the folk traditions of many cultures, as well as in many medical systems throughout the world. In contrast to this emphasis on individual health practices and habits of living, later physicians denied the healing power of nature and insisted that illness be treated quickly and aggressively.[14]

In a positive sense, the belief in the body's ability to heal itself means giving treatment which will boost its own healing mechanisms. The less aggressive the therapy, the less the potential there is for side effects. However, an alternative interpretation of the body's power to heal itself is an admission that the intervention of the practitioner may not be what causes the patient to get well. If the patient is suffering from a self-limiting condition which would have cured itself in a matter of time, it is probably unrealistic to claim that it was the therapy or the therapist which significantly contributed to the healing process. If the therapist is acting more as a medium through which self-healing occurs then this may shift the dynamics of the therapeutic relationship so that the actions of the patient become as important as the duties or obligations of the practitioner. This is an important shift from the doctor/patient relationship, in which the patient is viewed more often than not as the passive recipient of interventionist medical treatment. Accordingly, most bioethical theories focus on the actions of the practitioner as the moral agent, and not on the responsibilities of the patient. Similarly legal analysis of health care relationships places all of the responsibilities on the doctor and few, if any, on the patient. This may be inappropriate in analysing CAM relationships.

Emphasis on prevention rather than cure

CAM is as concerned with health maintenance and disease prevention as it is the removal of symptoms. As Fulder explains:

> [S]ome of the work of alternative medicine may be with people who are essentially symptom-free people. Alternative medicine deals not only with disease but also with vulnerabilities, concerning which it has a huge knowledge and catalogue of remedies. The skills of prevention and health maintenance rely on a concept of health in which many subtle levels of susceptibility and risk are regarded as states of health requiring assistance.[15]

The western focus on consulting doctors when ill is specific to our culture and times. Traditionally, in China, physicians were paid to keep patients sickness free. Patients would cease to pay if they became ill. Eisenberg explains that this is because the role of the classical Chinese physician, unlike that of most western doctors, was to teach patients to maximise health by living correctly. Since health and longevity, according to Chinese theory, depend not only on environment and genetics, but also on the patient's style of living, thoughts and emotions, the patient bears the primary responsibility for his of her health. Accordingly:

> Physicians did not fix broken bodies. They guided patients on personal quests for optimal physical and mental balance. This assistance came in the form of herbs, needles, massage and, above all, recommendations for behaviour modification.[16]

Appealing as such an approach may be, it is unlikely to find favour amongst western populations who are enculturated into consulting health care practitioners when they are sick. It does demonstrate that an ideal approach to health and healing would be closer to the World Health Organisation (WHO)'s definition of health than the ill health systems of the USA and Europe. Sometimes referred to as a utopian model of health, the WHO, in 1977, defined health as:

> A state of complete physical, mental, and social well-being, and not merely the absence of disease or infirmity.

Conventional medicine lacks the resources to aspire to such a far-reaching notion of health, especially in the world's poorest countries. Nonetheless, this definition at least offers an alternative version of the level of health to which people might aspire. It also recognises that healing is about more than curing patients' symptoms.

In determining whether a treatment has made a patient better, practitioners will want to look for both objective signs of improvement as well as the patient's subjective feelings on whether they feel better. Because CAM practitioners work with the body, mind and spirit, the patient's point of view becomes more important than when the treatment is designed merely to remove physical symptoms, which can be objectively ascertained. The absence, or reduction of morbidity is harder to ascertain than the presence of ill health. A huge ethical issue in CAM is how to measure the success or lack of success of the treatment. Whereas orthodox practitioners will tend to gauge this with reference to the alleviation of symptoms, the success of complementary treatment is that the patient stays well or does not have another episode of a recurrent illness. This can only be assessed after a period of time, and is a process operating along a continuum, rather than a single event. CAM practitioners tend not to think of patients as being absolutely well or absolutely ill. Many patients use CAM to remain symptom-free, and to experience an enhanced sense of well-being, which has implications for determining efficacy.

A further implication of CAM enhancing health, rather than dealing with ill health, is that the scope for treatment is limitless. There will be very few patients that a therapist need legitimately turn away, because therapists will always be able to do something, at some level, to enhance a patient's sense of well-being; often, it would seem, associated with the non-specific effects of the therapeutic interchange. What is currently lacking is the comparative data to show whether what the therapist can offer the patient is more likely to benefit the patient than any other intervention. Although some patients will choose to consult, say, an acupuncturist, or a homoeopath whatever their condition, other patients would like to be able to choose which practitioner they consult on the basis of sound evidence about whether a particular therapy is helpful for their condition.

If CAM is to become more closely integrated with conventional medicine, this difference in approach will have to be factored in by policy-makers and purchasers, who are more concerned both with efficacy and cost-effectiveness. In the present political climate, providers and third party insurers are unlikely to extend coverage to treatment of patients' vulnerabilities or susceptibilities.

Non-materialism

Conventional medicine concentrates its efforts on the material body, actively distancing itself from religion and superstition in favour of science. The centrality of materialism accounts for biomedicine's preoccupation with therapeutic interventions which cause obvious, measurable reactions in the physical body. Doctors have (begrudgingly) begun to accept the notion of a psychosocial body, although orthodox treatment is more commonly directed at removing physical symptoms.

The materialist world view is starkly at odds with the belief systems underpinning many alternative approaches to health and healing, which embrace non-material causes of ill health, and rely on non-materialistic concepts such as 'vital spirit', 'chi' or 'Qi' (vital energy) or 'prana' (life force). The difference between these two world views has important ramifications for the theory and politics of health. As Cassidy explains:

> One can only deliver care in a fashion which does not conflict with one's beliefs. If one accepts as real only what one can see, hear or measure with machines, then delivering care to the non-material bodies is, at the very least, puzzling.[17]

The difference between materialist conventional medicine and non-materialist alternative forms of belief systems are hard to reconcile, and are likely to hinder attempts at integration of conventional and non-conventional medicine. Materialists view alternative therapists with disdain because they fear that practitioners are more able to dupe patients, by purporting to work at a subtle energy level, the effects of which may not be readily ascertainable. Or, at best, they would argue that if CAM practitioners do treat patients successfully, this is wholly or largely due to the placebo effect. This has been defined as:

> a subjective improvement in the patient's condition that is not directly attributable to the pharmacological or physiological effects of treatment.[18]

This explanation overlooks the likelihood that the therapeutic relationship itself produces a placebo effect. Because the placebo effect consistently leads to improvements in about 35 per cent of patients, many therapists are keen to maximise and enhance this important self-healing response. In any event, materialists would argue that CAM patients may continue to receive 'treatment' when there is, in fact, very little physically wrong with them.

Non-materialists, in contrast, do not distinguish between 'real' (bodily) and 'imaginary' (emotional or spiritual) pain expressed by patients, rather viewing each as an expression of malfunctioning at different levels. At the same time, they are critical of the biomedical model and its preoccupation with the physical body and the removal of physical symptoms. Yet the emphasis in CAM on emotional and spiritual pain, may, inadvertently serve to further medicalise people's everyday problems and crises into something which can be 'treated', especially in first world countries where capitalist excess is manifesting an increasing sense of emotional and spiritual malaise.

Tendency to treat chronic rather than acute conditions

Studies suggest that CAM is most frequently used by patients suffering from chronic, rather than acute conditions. The 1997 follow-up survey conducted by Eisenberg *et al.* found that CAM approaches are most frequently used for back problems, anxiety, depression and headaches.[19] Different ethical tensions may arise in therapeutic relationships which work mostly with chronic conditions, rather than acute conditions. Some of the differences might include the following:

- It is rare for the treatment of chronic conditions to give rise to life or death ethical dilemmas. Breaches of confidentiality or abuses of professional boundaries are just as injurious to individual patients but are not given as much attention by the media.
- Treatment is not essential, in that the problem is not life-threatening, but the treatment, if successful, may significantly enhance the patient's quality of life. It might be argued that if patients have a 'right to life', this includes the right to a decent quality of life. As such, it may be possible to argue that CAM treatments are a legitimate health need, which ought to be considered more favourably in rationing debates.
- The patient will hopefully find the therapeutic encounter a positive experience. A massage or reflexology treatment is far more likely to be an enjoyable experience for a patient with frozen shoulder than receiving an injection of hydrocortisone. The enjoyment factor is likely to figure significantly in the patient's subjective interpretation of whether the therapeutic encounter was 'successful'.
- A patient suffering from a chronic condition will probably (but not always) be in a more robust position, mentally and physically, to make health care decisions, than patients in an acute condition. Accordingly, patients consulting CAM therapists need to have access to good quality

information, including information about the risks of treatment in order to make effective choices.

- The reductionist nature of modern western medicine means that for any diagnosed condition, there will usually be a specialist, or specialists, who deal with that problem or that part of the body. Holistic medicine would view regarding the body in such a way as anathema. The difficulty for patients trying to find the most appropriate therapist to deal with a chronic condition is that all therapies and therapists can legitimately claim to be able to do something to help. Once again, the question of who to consult becomes problematic.

A young woman in her early thirties is concerned that she is lacking in energy and feels lethargic and tired all of the time. In the past year, she has visited a reflexologist, a Reiki practitioner and an aromatherapist, each of whom attribute her tiredness to stress at work. Although she has felt 'lifted' for a short while after these sessions, the benefits are short-lived. On a friend's recommendation, she consults a naturopath. The naturopath suspects that the she is anaemic, and recommends that she asks her GP to do a blood test. The test confirms that the patient is anaemic and the naturopath advises her on how to increase the amount of iron in her diet. The patient is very pleased that she feels much more energetic, but is cross that none of the other practitioners she consulted were able to discover the problem earlier.

This example highlights a common problem for CAM practitioners who are keen to work holistically. A patient's symptoms might be attributed to psychological factors, when there is a simple physiological explanation. As well as highlighting the need for practitioners to know something about conventional diagnosis, it shows the difficulty patients face when they have a chronic problem which all practitioners claim they can do something for.

Charismatic teaching rather than externally accredited training

Whereas conventional medicine rests its foundations upon the edifice of rational science, many CAM therapies were borne out of the visionary ideas of a single practitioner, who has created a therapy and a body of knowledge. Classical homoeopathy, for example, was founded on the work of Samuel Hannehman and much of the teaching within classical homoeopathy is still based on Hannehman's original principles and findings. Similarly, modern osteopathy and chiropractic were developed by single individuals. These therapies may be contrasted with more ancient healing traditions which are often grounded in religions and traditions. These longer standing therapies may be equally hard to reconcile with conventional medical thinking, but do, at least, have the advantage of an empirical base, which has been built upon over thousands of years.

A striking feature of both of these sets of therapies is that they have often been taught, or passed on by charismatic personalities, who have attracted followers who have passed down the teachings of the masters, often relying on oral, rather than written traditions. Whilst valued by some consumers for their authenticity, this charismatic or self-styled approach to knowledge and its transmission is antithetical to modernist medicine. Over the last ten to fifteen years, the dominant CAM professionals have been aware that they need to bring their knowledge base and their educational processes closer into line with mainstream educational thinking and practice. The shift from charismatic teaching to more formalised systems of knowledge transmission coincides with the desire of a therapy to seek external validity and not just to impress its own members.[20] Where therapies are tied to the teaching and practice of a single individual, the therapy may have dedicated practitioners and adherents, but is unlikely to have much external credibility.

CAM therapists protest that traditional knowledge bases and alternative modes of knowledge acquisition should not be considered as inferior just because they run counter to current western educational policies. Degrees and diplomas may be sound educational vehicles for transmitting certain kinds of knowledge, but may be completely inappropriate in other areas, such as healing or traditional herbal medicine. Currently, it is assumed that a combined classroom and clinical approach to education is necessary to train health professionals and that knowledge skills and attitudes need to be kept up to date with regular and appropriate continuing professional development (CPD). Thus, at the same time as there has been a proliferation of diploma and degree courses for CAM therapists, there has been a concomitant rise in the availability of CPD courses.

This formalised approach to training will almost certainly be a requirement for therapies attempting to integrate with biomedicine. But we should not lose sight of the fact that there are other forms of knowledge, and other ways of knowing, which may be more appropriate to certain healing practices and which cannot be formalised into a three-year curriculum, leading to a licence to practise. Traditional healing systems recognise the value of an apprenticeship model of training in which the trainee's master decides, together with the new practitioner, when it is appropriate for the novice to see patients independently. Often, indigenous healers are chosen by the community elders at an early age, and spend many years learning their craft. Gutmanis describes how a native Hawaiian healer, or *Kahuna La'au Lapa'au*, would be trained:

> No matter when the novice began his training it was on the one-to-one relationship of a strict apprenticeship.... Never questioning, always observing, the boy began his training doing menial tasks....

There was a well established order of learning in the curriculum, but no set time of completion.[21]

Although this approach is uncommon in CAM, it may be an equally legitimate method of ensuring safe practice. These issues will be picked up again in Part II in the discussion of competence to practise, but for now it is essential that we do not assume that alternative traditions can be categorised and reproduced in a form which makes them more palatable to western consumers.

Ethically, the interesting issue is how far external credibility should count for more than patients' credibility. This debate extends beyond such formalistic questions as whether the colleges of such therapies have been externally accredited, and whether objective outcome measures can be demonstrated to support patients' enthusiastic testimonials. Rather, it touches upon the rights of individuals to reject the dominant paradigm and choose genuinely alternative approaches to dealing with their health. This turns on whether governments should adopt a broadly consumer freedom-based model or a consumer protection-based model.

Health care has always been an intensely regulated activity. Whether by direct methods of governance or by more distant means, modern states try to ensure that patients make wise health choices. This is likely to involve the licensing of practitioners and the licensing of therapeutic products. It is unlikely that people will be prevented from accessing such therapies – unless they represent such an obvious danger to health as to require external regulation. It is similarly unlikely that any state health provider or insurance will pay for a therapy the theoretical base of which turns upon the teachings of a single individual. Even therapies lacking external validation still need to be aware of ethical issues. Indeed, the need for ethical awareness is even greater amongst therapies which operate on the margins, since these practitioners are less likely to be subject to external forms of control.

Use of indigenous healing systems by ethnic communities

Modern health practitioners treat increasingly diverse patient populations. Recent and political unrest has led to mass displacement of whole populations, increasing the ethnic diversity of most westernised countries. This is presenting a host of issues for health care practitioners already inadequately trained to cope with the multi-cultural aspects of their work and the diverse ethnic and cultural background of their patients. The need to deliver culturally sensitive health care is an important aspect of competence and respect for autonomy and is no less so for CAM practitioners than it is for conventional health care practitioners.

Many cultures rely on indigenous forms of healing in place of conventional medicine. The use of certain traditional therapies, such as Ayurveda,

Navajo medicine, Tibetan medicine, Unani, shamanism and Traditional Chinese Medicine (TCM) is particularly high within ethnic communities. The right to pursue traditional approaches to health is an integral part of these communities' cultural heritage and belief systems. Many people in Britain turn to Ayurvedic practitioners or hakims before consulting a GP. To deprive communities access to the healing systems of their choice would be an infringement of their civil rights and personal freedoms.

Colonisation and integration into other cultures has meant that many groups have had to abandon their traditional healing methods. The self-determination movements taking hold in New Zealand, South Africa, Australia and Hawaii highlight access to indigenous healing as an important aspect of self-governance and cultural freedom. There, the question is not merely the right of all people to access treatment which they feel is congruent with their cultural beliefs, but the extent to which there should be government coverage of indigenous healing within mainstream funding. This question is particularly acute for cultures that have struggled to preserve and maintain traditional customs and health care practices post-colonisation. Should the New Zealand government support the integration of Maori healers into their existing health care coverage? Should US health insurers reimburse patients for use of Navajo medicine as well as more accepted CAM modalities, and if so, what criteria should be applied? It is unlikely that government funding will be forthcoming unless these indigenous methods can be shown, using whatever means appropriate, to be beneficial and not to cause harm.

Whilst these issues form part of the larger political debates around self-determination and restorative justice, distinct transcultural ethical issues arise. Is it legitimate for governments to demand that traditional indigenous healers demonstrate competence within a biomedical framework? How can the customs and beliefs underpinning indigenous healing systems be integrated into health care systems predicated on singularly western concepts of health and disease? If these healing practices are funded through central government resources, should they be offered first to native peoples and only then, subject to availability, to the rest of the population? Do these therapies work as effectively in non-indigenous populations?

Calls for respect to be shown towards alternative belief systems are not new. Patel,[22] considering the issue of integration in the USA, quotes Benjamin Rush, MD, Signatory of the Declaration of Independence and Physician to George Washington, who said, in relation to freedom of choice:

> The constitution of this Republic should make special provision for medical Freedom as well as Religious Freedom.... To restrict the art of healing to one class of men and deny equal privileges to others

will constitute the Bastille of medical science. All such laws are un-American and despotic.

Whilst traditional healing systems may not be provided within western conventional health care settings, their use, particularly within indigenous populations, is largely tolerated. Nonetheless, regulatory authorities are charged with a duty to protect all citizens from harm. The question for regulators remains whether indigenous healing practices represent an unacceptable risk of harm to people who avail themselves of them. This is a question which will be viewed very differently in countries where the bulk of the population has access to western conventional medicine and does not depend on traditional healing practices, and where diversity is more likely to be tolerated as an economic necessity.

How does this impact on CAM and indigenous healing practices? The history of CAM and indigenous healing is one of exclusion, based largely on its otherness in relation to the dominant paradigm of biomedicine. It would represent the worst sort of cultural imperialism to reject healing customs and practices merely because they are different to those of western medicine. It is, however, a legitimate ethical question to ask whether there should be controls over indigenous healing practices which can be used to good effect as well as bad, or whether health carers, whatever their background, ought to be able to satisfy core competencies aimed at assuring patient safety.

The freedom to choose the healing system of one's choice carries issues not just of individual liberty, but of cultural and ethnic identity. Even if indigenous healing practices were to be outlawed, they would continue to flourish underground. This is a clear example of the limits of formal governance, since ethnic communities will continue to value and utilise indigenous healing methods whatever their regulatory status. If this is the case, there is an additional imperative to provide resources, and facilitate research, to make these healing systems as safe as possible. Conventional doctors and nurses need to become more familiar with the healing practices their patients are likely to access and to discuss any possible areas of interaction. This applies to the use of indigenous healing systems as much as it does to the use of CAM.

Patients' different expectations of CAM

Having explored some of the shared characteristics of CAM, it is instructive to consider patients' expectations of CAM. CAM provides many functions in society. It is not solely concerned with removing manifestations of physical ill health. This will inevitably impact on any analysis of the ethics of the CAM relationship. For some patients, their relationship with a CAM therapist is much more akin to a psychotherapeutic relationship than a 'medical' relationship. CAM relationships may be about managing a particular health episode, but may simultaneously be about helping a patient to achieve longer term autonomy and control over their well-being and destiny. The fact that in many cases patients actively *enjoy* these therapeutic encounters also influences the ethical obligations of both patient and practitioner.

What then, are some of the motivations for patients seeking CAM therapy? Who seeks out CAM therapy and why? Unsurprisingly, there is no such thing as a typical CAM patient. The stereotype that CAM is used predominantly by middle aged, middle-class women no longer holds true, notwithstanding evidence that women access health care more often than men, and the inference that patients must have a certain level of financial flexibility if they are paying for CAM encounters out of their own pockets. The following suggestions represent some possible motivations for a patient's decision to pursue CAM:

- Because conventional medical medicine has failed them in the past, or because they feel that the level of side effects from conventional treatment is unacceptable.
- Because they do not want to discuss this particular problem/(s) with their GP/conventional physician, perhaps because they find CAM therapists more sympathetic.
- Because they are looking for an explanation of their illness in spiritual or emotional, rather than scientific, terms.
- Because they know of other people who have sought CAM and been impressed with the results.
- Because their conventional physician has recommended CAM.
- Because they view CAM, on some level, as an alternative to psychotherapy and welcome the opportunity 'to be heard' by a caring individual.
- In the case of 'hands-on' therapies, because they value the physical contact that the therapy offers.
- Because alternative medicine is more congruent with beliefs in other areas of their life, such as concern for the environment or disdain for pharmaceutical-driven western medicine.
- Because they wish to avoid ill health in the future and see CAM as a way of promoting or enhancing their well-being.
- Because CAM is currently considered to be fashionable and is branded as a consumer product, leading patients to view CAM in similar terms to leisure or entertainment

Much debate has focussed on the difference between therapists who work in a 'complementary' fashion, that is, alongside conventional doctors, and 'alternative' practitioners, who offer a genuine substitute. This semantic debate does not seem to represent the manner in which most patients utilise different healing systems, viewing complementary, alternative and allopathic as options which are all at their disposal and available to be used concurrently.

Greater ethical concerns have been voiced in relation to alternative practitioners who provide a 'complete system' of healing, because these therapists are more likely to diagnose and treat within a genuinely alternative paradigm and are thought to be more likely to dissuade patients from seeking conventional approaches from which they might benefit. Accordingly, the codes of many complementary therapists stress that practitioners are not medical doctors and should not 'diagnose' the patient. This is unrealistic because every therapist must diagnose in the sense of listening to the patient's story, making observations and coming to a decision as to what form of treatment to provide.

It is clear that not all patients who consult CAM practitioners are 'ill', or consider themselves as 'patients' in the conventional sense. Bioethics, for the main part, rarely questions the presumption that patients are ill and that the practitioner's job is 'to make them better'. The focus of ethical interest is invariably on the moral responsibilities of the health professional as the significant moral agent, and not on those of the patient, seen merely as the passive moral subject. The ethics of 'ill health' medicine may differ in vital respects from the ethics of 'wellness-medicine'. CAM patients seeking to enhance their well-being, or balance their 'chi' may be seeking a service from a practitioner as a consumer and view themselves as on a par with the practitioner rather than seeing themselves as a dependent, sick, vulnerable patient.

This has relevance if one considers Eisenberg et al.'s findings that more than half of all encounters in the USA with CAM therapists are with chiropractors and massage therapists.[23] Whereas consultations with chiropractors may give rise to ethical issues similar to those encountered in the doctor/patient relationship, the motivations of people seeking massage therapy may have little to do with treating an illness. Massage therapy is a good example of a CAM therapy in which the client may not regard himself or herself as a patient and may view the therapeutic encounter more as an aspect of leisure than health care. Traditionally, people are thought to be free to engage in whatever leisure activities they please, however extreme; the risk being up to the individual. In such a situation, the responsibility lies primarily with the individual person to choose the practitioner who best meets his/her requirements.

Rather than posing the question: 'What are the ethical responsibilities of CAM therapists', an alternative way of framing the discussion is to ask what are the expectations of this particular CAM client and are they being met? Most ethical tensions within a therapeutic encounter arise because of a mismatch between the patient's expectations and what the practitioner delivers. I have suggested above that the reasons people consult CAM practitioners may be far more complex than simply because they are ill. If CAM relationships are truly patient-centred, then every therapist should endeavour to ascertain what the particular patient hopes to gain out of therapy, since this will direct the course of the therapeutic encounter. Ethical tensions are far less likely to arise where there is congruence between what the patient wants and what the patient gets. Patients' needs may be 'health' related or not, depending, in no small part, on how narrowly or broadly one defines 'health'.

Patients do not seem to want a scientific explanation for their illness when they consult a CAM practitioner, nor do they seem to want a scientific explanation for how the therapy works. Rather, some patients seem to be looking for a non-materialist, non-reductionist explanation for their malaise. According to Vickers and Zollman:

> Complementary practitioners may have explanations that make sense to patients such as describing illness as a result of environmental factors or as a physical expression of emotional patterns. Conventional medicine may have problems with such explanations if they have no scientific justification, but sociological research shows that patients consider them beneficial when they reinforce their own beliefs and expectations.[24]

It is worth therapists thinking seriously about what and who is driving the research agenda, and what research is important. Some CAM practitioners are keen to understand how their modality works, yet other practitioners are content to treat without this knowledge. The current limited evidence-base for CAM has not hindered its growth so far, but, it will be argued, may do so in the future. As CAM therapies rush towards professionalisation, it is worth therapists reflecting on the alternative nature and origins of their therapy and whether support for the therapy lies in the very differences that integration would probably seek to obliterate.

The political context of CAM

The ethical implications of CAM cannot be divorced from the political context in which it operates. Health has never been higher on the political agenda. The provision of high quality, affordable, health care is a huge voting issue. The availability of CAM raises fundamental political questions including:

- How far do democratically elected governments have a responsibility to provide health care which is responsive to consumers' preferences?
- Should governments seek to prevent people from making ill-informed health choices or should individuals who are paying for CAM therapies themselves be free to negotiate terms as they see fit?

- Should governments seek to regulate health-related phenomena, including indigenous healing rituals, which are more akin to religion, and which are at odds with secular tradition and concepts of health and disease?
- Can governments be neutral in their dealings with CAM when they receive so much revenue from pharmaceutical companies?

Governments clearly have a vested interest in the health of their nations. In industrialised societies, this interest is predominantly economic, tied in with the need to have a healthy work force. It is probably not coincidental that research funding has been made available to establish the efficacy of chiropractic, given the number of days of work lost each year through people suffering from lower back pain. Regulation, in most spheres of activity, is geared, directly or indirectly, towards ensuring that people are able to work, to produce and to consume.

The scope of CAM therapists to practise and CAM patients to receive CAM therapies is largely dependent on how governments view these therapies as fitting in with overall health strategies. In this regard, changing political climates have a direct impact on the practice of CAM. A free market economy stressing decentralisation and deregulation is unlikely to impose excessive restraints on which therapies are offered and how they are regulated. In terms of health, governments which are trying to reduce dependence upon the state, and foster a sense of independence and self-reliance, may look favourably on complementary therapies which promote self-healing and taking personal responsibility for one's health and well-being.

However, governments which have previously adopted a *laissez-faire* approach towards CAM may feel compelled to take a more interventionist stance if new trends emerge. These might include evidence showing that patients are being harmed by CAM, CAM expanding beyond its present boundaries and offering a viable alternative to seriously ill patients, or CAM growing to such an extent that it becomes a significant economic threat to drug-based conventional medicine.

What is the current political state of play? This is hard to assess, because the political status of CAM is dynamic and in a constant state of flux. In the UK, a recent report by the House of Lords Select Committee on Science and Technology was broadly favourable towards CAM, whilst calling for more research, consistently high training standards, better regulation and a commitment towards evidence-based practice.[25] Their Lordships and the government were critical of the proliferation of professional bodies within the same therapy and strongly urged therapies to come together under a single, registering body. They regarded this as essential to improving standards of training and practice. The UK government has endorsed the main recommendations of the Select Committee's report, reinforcing the need for a stronger evidence base as a precursor to integration.

Because the existence and success of CAM impacts so obviously on vested interests of the medical establishment and pharmaceutical industry, governments' motives and strategies for decision-making are rarely transparent. Certain trends are discernible nonetheless, and an important political marker is the interface between CAM and orthodox medicine. Undoubtedly, the relationship between CAM and orthodox medicine has changed dramatically since the 1990s. Increasingly, more and more doctors accept that complementary and alternative therapies have a useful role to play in the treatment of certain conditions. In the preface to their book, *Complementary/Alternative Medicine. An Evidence-Based Approach*, Spencer and Jacobs draw attention to the intensity of the debate surrounding the creation of the Office of Alternative Medicine (OAM) at the National Institutes of Health (NIH) in the United States, noting that:

> at the centre of this debate was whether CAM could or should be evaluated because of past perceptions of mysticism and outright frauds.[26]

The softening of the medical profession's attitudes towards CAM was evident in the British Medical Association's 1993 publication: *Complementary Medicine: New Approaches to Good Practice*, which supported the use of complementary medicine provided practitioners were sufficiently well trained and accountable to professional bodies.[27] Currently in both the UK and the USA, significant proportions of medical and nursing schools are offering students courses in CAM familiarisation, or in some cases, the basics of CAM therapeutics. Growing numbers of health insurers are demonstrating a greater willingness to reimburse patients for certain therapies, although the extent to which they are prepared to do this varies enormously, and may be restricted to referrals by a GP/primary health physician. Symbolically, the UK government is now providing a small amount of money for research in CAM, and medical charities and other funding institutions have expressed interest in funding well-designed CAM research projects.

Slowly, but surely, the ground is shifting. Although some doctors remain implacably opposed to complementary and alternative therapies, the gulf between conventional and alternative approaches is narrowing. As more is known about psycho-social impact on physical health, conventional doctors are becoming more responsive to the need to treat patients holistically. Although conventional medicine has been highly successful in reducing mortality and morbidity in certain clinical areas, most doctors accept that conventional medicine fails patients with chronic, intractable conditions. There is also growing societal concern about the costs of high-tech medicine, both in financial terms, and in terms of side effects of modern medicines, including the re-emergence of epidemics due to overuse of antibiotics. These factors have allowed CAM to flourish to an unprecedented extent.

However, there is a price to pay for this shift in attitude. Cynics warn against the change in nomenclature from 'fringe' medicine in the 1960s, to 'alternative' in the 1970s and 1980s and 'complementary' in the 1990s, to talk of 'integrated medicine' as the medicine for the millennium. Many CAM practitioners fear that the moves towards 'integration' is misguided, because it presupposes integration of CAM into conventional medicine, and this will result in a medical take-over, or 'colonisation', rather than a truly collaborative venture.

As more conventional practitioners express an interest in making CAM therapies available to their patients and undertake short courses in CAM therapies, 'lay' practitioners fear that there is a strong chance that doctors will 'cherry pick' those interventions which can be shown to work in repro- ducible studies and will offer CAM to patients in medicalised settings. The proliferation of courses targeted at doctors, nurses, physiotherapists and other professions allied to medicine is doing little to allay these fears. An increased availability of CAM within conventional settings may prove to be counter-productive, given that patient satisfaction has been linked to the time available for the consultation, the more relaxed atmosphere in which CAM consultations tend to take place, and the non-reductionist, holistic approach which CAM therapists offer. It is unlikely that this could be repli- cated in a hospital or clinic. But patients may, increasingly, be prepared to accept a watered-down version of CAM, if it were offered to them free, or covered by their health insurance.

Wide-scale integration of CAM and conventional medicine is unlikely until a stronger evidence base exists. In the absence of a strong scientific research tradition within CAM, much of the current research into comple- mentary medicine is being carried out by conventional doctors. This is further fuelling concerns of lay practitioners that CAM, if not regulated out of existence, will become medicalised and reduced to a set of clinical inter- ventions rather than an entire philosophical tradition. The research issue is a deeply political area, with little money invested in areas which cannot yield profit. The impetus for researching CAM approaches is that they may prove to be less costly in the long run than conventional medical alternatives.

Conclusion

CAM is political because health and health care is political. The ethics of CAM cannot be divorced from the politics of CAM. Practitioners might want to reflect on whether the factors which have permitted CAM to flourish in recent years indicate a radical redefinition of health or a passing trend. Ironically, CAM might now be considered a victim of its own success. By virtue of its size it can no longer be regarded as 'fringe' or 'marginal'. CAM is now big business, providing many patients with a viable alternative to conventional medicine. At a time of increased consumer sophistication, patients can be as critical of complementary and alternative therapists as they are of doctors. Patients who are paying for their health care expect value for money, and will want to know which therapy is most likely to benefit them and why.

To maintain current levels of enthusiasm, CAM practitioners will need to be able to give consumers a reason for investing in their services. In the past, therapists have often traded on their ability to spend more time with patients than doctors can, and to treat the 'whole patient'. But however much patients value these aspects of the therapeutic encounter, they will only continue to use, or return to, complementary and alternative therapists for further ailments if, in addition to their empathy, therapists are also able to deliver favourable health outcomes. The days of blind faith are disappearing fast, and CAM practitioners, like their conventional medical counterparts, need to establish a credible basis if they are to sustain consumer confidence.

Much enthusiasm for CAM has been generated through the successful deployment of various marketing strategies, portraying complementary and alternative therapists as 'patient-centred'. The media generally portray CAM as safe, implying that 'nature's remedies' means 'gentle' and 'free from harmful side effects'. Product manufacturers are also keen to make this link. The term 'alternative approach' is usually conflated with a 'holistic approach'. Whilst there may be some truth in these labels, being 'green' or 'patient-centred' is of little value if the therapy is not efficacious. Many alternative practitioners do not work holistically (whilst many conventional practitioners sincerely endeavour to do so), and it is increasingly known that most therapies carry side effects ranging from minor to severe. In the UK, a coroner attributed a man's death to osteopathic treatment given for tennis elbow received shortly before he died. A number of herbal remedies are extremely toxic, and the UK government is currently attempting to prohibit the use of the Chinese herb *Aristolochia*, which has been lined to cancer of the urinary system.[28] In 1994, thirty women in Belgium suffered severe kidney damage after taking a slimming remedy accidentally containing this herb, as well as two other Chinese herbs, *S tetandra* and *Magnolia officinalis*.

Responsible practitioners never overstate their ability to help individual clients, and any therapist who guarantees a cure is inviting dissatisfaction (if not prosecution under the relevant consumer legislation). Any intervention which has the capacity to benefit, also has the capacity to cause harm. The side effects of CAM treatment may be psychological as well as physical. Patients need to be warned of the risks of CAM just as much as they do the risks of conventional treatments. Similarly, practitioners need to accept that in certain situations, the best treatment to give the patient is no treatment at all – a challenging proposition for private practitioners struggling to make a living.

This book will consider the ethical implications for CAM at this time of political flux. The ethical basis of the patient/practitioner relationship must be seen as being at the heart of the therapeutic encounter. Whilst political and regulatory forces change from one year to the next, the fundamental responsibility to benefit and not harm has remained the cornerstone of therapeutic practice for thousands of years and remains the basis of all forms of medicine in the new millennium.

Notes

1 This point is explored by Coope, C.M. (1996) 'Does Teaching By Cases Mislead Us About Morality?'. *Journal of Medical Ethics.* 22: 46–52.
2 *The Chantilly Report: Alternative Medicine; Expanding Medical Horizons* (1992). A Report to the National Institutes of Health on Alternative Medical Systems and Practices in the United States.
3 Eisenberg, D.M., Davis, R.B., Ettner, S.I., *et al.* (1998) 'Trends in Alternative Medicine Use in the United States, 1990–1997: Results of a Follow-up National Survey'. *Journal of the American Medical Association.* 280: 1569–1575.
4 Wetzel, M.S., Eisenberg, D.M. and Kaptchuk, T.J. (1988) 'Courses Involving Complementary and Alternative Medicine at US Medical Schools'. *Journal of the American Medical Association.* 280: 784–787.
5 Eskinazi, D. (1998) 'Factors that Shape Alternative Medicine'. *Journal of the American Medical Association.* 280(18), November 11.
6 Sharma, U. (1992) *Complementary Medicine Today: Practitioners and Patients.* Tavistock, Routledge: London and New York.
7 Douglas, M. (1994) 'The Construction of the Physician. A Cultural Approach to Medical Fashions'. In Budd, S. and Sharma, U. (eds) *The Healing Bond.* Routledge: London and New York.
8 Cohen, M. (1998) *Complementary and Alternative Medicine: Legal Boundaries and Regulatory Perspectives.* Johns Hopkins University Press: Baltimore, MD and London.
9 Fulder, S. (1988) 'The Basic Concepts of Alternative Medicine and Their Impact on Our Views of Health'. *The Journal of Alternative and Complementary Medicine.* 4(2): 147–158.
10 Kottow, M. (1992) 'Classical Medicine v Alternative Medical Practices'. *Journal of Medical Ethics.* 18: 18–22.
11 Fulder, op. cit.
12 Kottow, op. cit.
13 Micozzi, M. (ed.) (1996) *Fundamentals of Complementary and Alternative Medicine.* Churchill Livingstone: Edinburgh.
14 Lipson, J. and Steiger, N. (1996) *Self-Care Nursing in a Multicultural Context.* Sage: Thousand Oaks, CA, London and New Delhi.
15 Fulder, op. cit.
16 Eisenberg, D. with Wright, T.L. (1995) *Encounters with Qi. Exploring Chinese Medicine.* W.W. Norton & Co., Inc.: New York.
17 Cassidy, C.M. (1996) 'Cultural Context of Complementary and Alternative Medicine Systems'. In Micozzi, M. (ed.), op. cit.
18 Lewith, G.T. (1993) 'Every Doctor a Walking Placebo'. In Lewith, G.T. and Aldridge, D. (eds) *Clinical Research Methodology for Complementary Therapies.* Hodder and Stoughton: Sevenoaks.
19 Eisenberg D.M., *et al.*, op. cit.
20 Cant, S. and Sharma, U. (eds) (1996) *Complementary and Alternative Medicines. Knowledge in Practice.* Free Association Books Ltd: London.

21 Gutmanis, J. (1999) *Kahuna La'au Lapa'au. The Practice of Hawaiian Herbal Medicine*. Island Heritage Publishing: Norfolk Island.
22 Patel, V. (1988) 'Understanding the Integration of Alternative Modalities into an Emerging Health Care Model in the United States'. In Humber, J. and Almeder, R. (eds) *Alternative Medicine and Ethics*. Humana Press: Totowa, NJ.
23 Eisenberg D.M., *et. al.*, op. cit.
24 Vickers, A. and Zollman, C. (1999) 'ABC of Complementary Medicine. Complementary Medicine and the Patient'. *British Medical Journal.* 319:1486–1489.
25 House of Lords. Sixth Report of the House of Lords Science and Technology Committee (2000) *Complementary and Alternative Medicine*. London: The Stationery Office.
26 Spencer, J.W. and Jacobs, J.J. (eds) (1999) *Complementary/Alternative Medicine. An Evidence-Based Approach*. Mosby: St Louis, MO.
27 British Medical Association (1993) *Complementary Medicine: New Approaches to Good Practice*. British Medical Association and Oxford University Press: London and Oxford.
28 Gottlieb, S. (2000) 'Chinese Herb May Cause Cancer'. *British Medical Journal.* 320: 1623.

Part I

UNDERSTANDING ETHICS

2

WHAT DO WE MEAN
BY 'ETHICS'?

The interest in health care ethics over the last thirty years reflects many of the same cultural shifts which account for the increased attraction of non-conventional therapies. There has been a general disillusionment with authority and a refusal to accept the view of 'the experts'. At the same time, there has been a growth of interest in consumer rights. These social changes have prompted dramatic shifts in the relationship between patients and their conventional health practitioners. In the past, patients accepted doctors' advice uncritically. They are now expected to explain the available options to their patients and are required by law to provide sufficient information to enable the patient to choose whether to accept or refuse treatment. This is most notably witnessed in the transformation of the doctor/patient relationship from a model of benign paternalism to a therapeutic alliance in which informed patients are encouraged to participate in decision-making.

During this time, there has been a dramatic ethical shift from a model of health care ethics which had been virtually unchanged since Hippocrates, in which the beneficent physician ministered to the sick, towards a model in which respecting the patient's autonomy has come to be viewed as an integral aspect of benefiting them. This has been translated into law through the requirement of obtaining informed consent to treatment. In the USA and the UK, there is now a presumption that, other than in the case of emergencies, treatment should not be given unless the patient has been adequately informed about the risks involved in the treatment and any alternatives to the treatment (including no treatment at all) and the patient has agreed to the treatment.

The consent requirement is not just about being sued. Rather, it is recognition that respecting the patient's autonomy is an intrinsic part of being a 'good' practitioner. Health choices should be the patient's, guided by the practitioner. Although the doctor may be the technical expert, patients are the experts when it comes to their own bodies, their fears and desires. To give an example, a doctor may feel that a hysterectomy is the best medical treatment to control a female patient's excessive menstrual bleeding, whereas the psychological implications for that woman may preclude such a drastic option. In the past, the notion of medical paternalism may have supported doctors who bullied women into accepting the 'medically' appropriate treatment. Now, a doctor who performs a hysterectomy without consent is likely to be sued for assault and struck off. Even in such extreme cases, it is worth noting that doctors rarely act out of malevolence, but out of a mistaken belief that they know what is in the patient's best interests.

This reconfiguring of the therapeutic encounter has been less evident within CAM, where greater patient involvement has always been more in evidence. Nevertheless, increased patient sophistication, combined with calls for greater accountability, have led many CAM practitioners to similarly re-evaluate the dynamics of their therapeutic relationships.

The focus of this book is to demonstrate why practising ethically is so important. The central proposition is that it is impossible to be a 'good' practitioner unless one is an ethical practitioner. Thinking about ethics is not something which a practitioner does after deciding what treatment the patient needs to be given, but is an integral part of how to relate to the patient. Health care practice involves people who, by reason of ill health, are more likely to be vulnerable and reliant upon others. Patients entrust highly personal information about themselves to a virtual stranger, they allow themselves to undergo intimate examination, and they submit to recommended treatment in the hope and desire that it will benefit them. In seeking the healing ministrations of another, they are tacitly admitting that they need help and are prepared to swap some of their autonomy for a period of dependence on someone who can heal them. It should be obvious that the corollary of this is that the health carer is in a position of considerable power. The health care relationship depends upon a high level of trust between the client and the therapist. The client has to take a leap of faith that the carer can be trusted to do only what is in the patient's interests and that the trust which has been placed in the carer will not be abused.

Most practitioners do not deliberately set out to abuse that position of trust. As in any occupational group there will always be a small percentage of practitioners who deliberately use their position of power in an abusive fashion. Such behaviour is abhorrent and should be subject to the most stringent legal penalties and professional disciplinary action. But the focus of this book is not extreme and rare cases of abuse, but the more widespread, and possibly even inadvertent, ethical abuses perpetrated by ordinary practitioners.

The scope of ethics is considerably wider than many therapists may at first realise. *Central to this thesis is the contention that therapists must have a sound basis for recommending that their therapy will be able to offer some benefit to the patient.* This key point goes much deeper than the perennial objection of hostile sectors of the medical profession that there is insufficient evidence to substantiate CAM therapies. It goes to the heart of whether therapists truly ask themselves what it is that their therapy can provide both for patients in general and for the particular patient in front of them. Until therapists can satisfactorily answer this fundamental question, their right to call themselves health professionals must be questioned.

What does it mean to practise ethically?

Practising ethically or morally means different things to different people. CAM practitioners have to resolve differences between the ethics or values of their profession, the values of their patients, and their personal values. No two practitioners will necessarily respond to an ethical dilemma in the same way, yet neither are necessarily 'right' or 'wrong'. The following examples illustrate dilemmas that might be encountered.

A chiropractor knows from past experience that if she explains to a patient what a high velocity thrust feels like before she does it, the patient is likely to become tense and stiffen up, so she tends to act first and explain later.

A homoeopath treating a fourteen-year-old girl for recurrent urinary tract infection is concerned that the girl is being abused by her stepfather but is unsure whether, or to whom, this information should be disclosed.

For six months, a medical herbalist has been treating a nineteen-year-old male suffering from mild depression. When the patient commits suicide, his family threaten to sue the therapist for failing to realise the severity of his condition.

A reflexologist who suspects that his patient has bowel cancer feels that the patient's spirits are so likely to be damaged by disclosing bad news that he keeps his opinion to himself.

An acupuncturist sees a new patient who is extremely critical of her former acupuncturist. Having listened to the patient's story, the acupuncturist is inclined to agree that the former acupuncturist, who happens to be a friend, has acted unprofessionally and possibly been negligent. The acupuncturist does not know whether to report her friend to their professional body.

An osteopath wishes to treat a patient using a combination of osteopathy, cranio-sacral therapy and acupuncture, but because of the wording of the patient's insurance policy, feels compelled to lie about both the nature of the treatment which will be provided and the length of time that the patient has been suffering from the condition requiring treatment.

In each situation, practitioners are having to make, or have made, a moral deliberation, deciding what is the right course of action and being able to justify why they have acted in this way. In each scenario, the problem is an ethical dilemma and not a technical problem. In each case, the practitioner, as a moral agent, has choices as to which course of action to take. Often, all available options are unpalatable. The homoeopath who suspects child abuse may feel that she is duty bound to report her suspicions to social services, even though this may result in the child being put into care and the break up of a family. To be a health professional is to make hard choices and to be accountable for them.

This section of the book concentrates on *how* therapists make moral decisions and what tools they can use to make the best ethical decision in the circumstances. Whereas some authors might favour a purely practical approach to this ethical decision-making, looking at real and hypothetical examples to explore the issues, any meaningful reflection on ethical dilemmas requires therapists to have some knowledge of the various theoretical bases for thinking about what it means to 'do the right thing', or at the very least, arriving at a decision which is morally justifiable. Only once ethical theories have been discussed can therapists begin to think reflectively about what it means to act ethically and how these ideas can be applied to dilemmas arising in their own practice.

What this book cannot do is provide practitioners with a step-by-step guide for how they ought to act in every potentially controversial situation. Abstract ethical theory can only take one so far. It would be unrealistic to pretend that psychological and political factors do not influence how practitioners choose to act. The highly individualised nature of CAM relationships means that much depends on the precise dynamic between the practitioner and the patient and the terms by which they have agreed to enter into a constructive therapeutic relationship. To attempt to provide practitioners with a universal set of answers ignores the context in which the problem has arisen, the relationship between the parties, and the motivations and values of the parties.

No-one can make ethical choices on behalf of a therapist and no-one other than the therapist will be held professionally accountable for the decisions which are made. Four basic principles, however, may help practitioners to understand what is involved in acting ethically, and will allow them to use the material in this book as a guide to practical decision-making. The essence of these principles is to remind practitioners that good practice demands attention to the ethical component of the therapeutic encounter. Making ethical decisions requires practitioners to be familiar with ethical theory and to acquire the skills of critical reflection to be able to apply theory to practice.

Principle one

Ethics is not solely about rare dramatic conflicts. It concerns all aspects of the therapeutic encounter, including the practitioner's competence, boundaries between the practitioner and patient, the patient's right to make decisions based on informed choices, respect for the patient's culture and values, and confidentiality. The fact that CAM rarely involves life or death decisions does not mean that there are fewer ethical issues in CAM therapeutic relationships. Any interaction with a patient (including a potential patient or a former patient) can give rise to ethical tensions.

Principle two

Ethical awareness is an ongoing process requiring active deliberation. Therapists can learn, through a process of reflection, how to apply a range of ethical theories to assist their decision-making and, indeed, have a moral duty to do so. Even though there may be no 'right answer' to a given dilemma, therapists have a moral responsibility to consider their options in the light of existing ethical theories, and to be sure that their decisions are ethically defensible and will stand up to external scrutiny. Since practitioners make most of their ethical decisions behind closed doors, practitioners must regulate their own conduct.

Principle three

Acting ethically requires a practitioner to be aware of all relevant professional codes and to know about any particular laws governing his or her sphere of practice, since these are additional mechanisms for regulating the individual therapist's conduct. The rules contained in codes of ethics represent standards of conduct which society expects professionals to follow. These may impose more onerous duties on health professionals than those which apply to ordinary members of the public, but to be a professional is a privilege, which confers both rights and responsibilities. The shortcomings of both ethical codes and law as a means of regulating the professional relationship make it all the more important that practitioners are aware of their ethical responsibilities, and become habituated to making good moral choices.

Principle four

Health care ethics involves benefiting patients and not causing them harm. Acting ethically requires practitioners to be aware of professional developments and research underpinning their therapy to ensure competence. It will rarely be ethical for therapists to work in complete isolation from their professional colleagues and with little regard for developments in their field.

In order to provide patients with a range of options, practitioners should be aware of developments in health and social care generally.

The bigger picture: can we agree on what is right or wrong?

How do we know whether our actions are right or wrong and whether we share a common understanding about what it means to act ethically? This involves asking where our ethical principles come from. Are they universal or God-given truths? Do ethical precepts apply absolutely or are they specific to different times and different cultures?

At the heart of this book is the question, 'How do practitioners know what is the right thing to do?' We might think that most people share a basic moral framework, but the polarisation generated by most ethical issues of the day reveal that this is simply not the case. Ethical deliberation cannot simply be a matter of allowing each practitioner to act according to his or her intuition, since on closer analysis, gut reactions vary enormously depending on a person's cultural background, socio-economic status, political beliefs, values, prejudices, personal history and the views of others who have shaped that person's moral development and education.

If this is so, is there anything which can be universally considered right, or does the answer always depend on the individual's standpoint? Is the right thing to do self-evident and universally agreed, entirely relative, or somewhere between the two? Philosophers have wrestled with this question for thousands of years and opinion is deeply divided on the subject. Many contemporary philosophers reject the idea of ethical moral relativity because this implies that all moral standpoints are equally acceptable, or 'anything goes'. Many people do seem to feel that some things are self-evidently right or wrong, but do not wish to appear insensitive to other people's cultural values and beliefs merely because they differ to their own.

The case for moral relativity

Moral relativists maintain that each community develops its own system of ethics to meet its own needs. The system which emerges is culturally and socially determined in light of the needs of that society at that point in time. Within certain indigenous cultures, it may be regarded as normal or appropriate to use prayer as a primary means of treating a seriously ill child, whereas in parts of the USA or the UK, failure to obtain conventional treatment constitutes child abuse.

The question of moral relativity is very pertinent to a discussion of CAM ethics, since many therapies are grounded in non-western philosophical traditions and do not share western concepts of health, the body, or individual autonomy. Neither the Chinese nor the Japanese culture approves of burdening sick individuals with choices about their own health, and both exhibit a level of paternalism which many western patients would find unacceptable. What influence will this have on a traditionally trained Chinese herbalist or a Japanese shiatsu practitioner? Can we expect that if they are working in the west they will automatically accept ethical theories which prioritise individual autonomy over the needs of the family or the community? What ethical system should be invoked when practitioners are treating patients whose cultural belief systems are very different to their own?

This question is also important because most therapists work in multicultural societies and treat patients from a variety of backgrounds. Therapists should not presume that their patients will experience concepts such as pain, illness, health, autonomy, suffering, quality of life, dying or childhood in the same way that they themselves do. Any ethical analysis must take this into account, because these cultural factors will impact on ethical issues such as when it is right to tell the truth or when it necessary to seek the patient's consent. In responding to different patients' health beliefs, practitioners must learn to synthesise their own position with those of their patients if they are to be able to offer an effective response. Cassidy argues:

> The practice of cultural relativity is pivotal to the study of alternative medicine, because each alternative system of medicine provides a different set of ideas about the body, disease and medical reality.[1]

Wong, a Chinese-American philosopher, argues that the reason moral relativism is usually rejected is because opponents draw on the most extreme examples, such as cannibalism, to argue that some things are universally or absolutely wrong. This is unhelpful, particularly when, as is usually the case, the example given is taken out of context. For example, reliance on prayer instead of conventional treatment makes more sense to ill people in traditional societies who believe that ancestors continue to protect the living, even after their death, or, conversely, may cause disease amongst the living.[2] This may seem irrational to health professionals, but the principle of respect for individual autonomy allows people to hold irrational beliefs and to refuse treatment on that basis, even if it will result in their death.[3]

Wong proposes that more than one moral viewpoint can be legitimate. The example he uses is particularly pertinent to our inquiry:

> One apparent and striking difference that would be a good candidate for this sort of argument concerns the emphasis on individual rights that is embodied in the ethical culture of the modern West and that seems absent in traditional cultures found in Africa, China, Japan and India. The content of duties in such traditional cultures instead seems organised around the central value of a

common good that consists in a certain sort of ideal community life, a network of relationships, partially defined by social roles, again, ideal, but imperfectly embodied in ongoing existing practice. The ideal for members is composed of various virtues that enable them, given their place in the network of relationships, to promote and sustain the common good.[4]

Within Confucianism, the family and kinship groups are models for the common good. This was reflected in political and, indeed, ethical practice, where benevolent leaders ruled with the aim of cultivating virtue and harmony among their subjects. In many traditional cultures, individuals find their happiness not through having their personal preferences continually satisfied, but in working towards the promotion of the common good. Where there is a fundamental harmony between the good of the individual and the common good, it would be reasonable to expect greater constraints on individual freedom than exist in traditions where there is no such harmony.[5] Wong uses these examples to argue that far from one or the other tradition being 'right', each tradition focusses on a good that may reasonably occupy the centre of an ethical ideal for human life:

> On the one hand, there is the good of belonging to and contributing to a community; on the other, there is the good of respect for the individual apart from any contribution to community. It would be surprising if there were just one justifiable way of setting a priority with respect to the two goods. It should not be surprising, after all, if the range of human goods is simply too rich and diverse to be reconciled in just a single moral ideal.[6]

The idea that different moral viewpoints co-exist has implications for CAM practice. Patients may have to accept that a practitioner who works from a different cultural perspective may provide care in ways the patient may not have imagined and may have a different style and professional ethos than a western health care practitioner. For example, traditionally trained acupuncturists might not always explain what points they are needling to the patient or why they have chosen those precise points. In an alternative healing consultation, there may be far less communication than the patient expects. Patients need to realise that when they consult a practitioner who works within a different philosophical framework, this will affect the therapeutic exchange. In some cases, the differences will be cosmetic, such as encouraging yoga students to close their practice with the Sanskrit word 'Namaste'. In other situations, the differences may be profound, for example, where a practitioner declines to discuss the treatment and evades questions because the practitioner feels these are not things the patient needs to know.

The case for universal ethics

Universalists believe that some things are absolutely right and others absolutely wrong. Unlike moral relativists, who believe that ethical standards are unique to the society they inhabit, universalists believe that ethical values are objective and eternal and do not rely on social acceptance for their validity. They take the view that moral values are permanent and fixed entities. In the past, universalists have subscribed to the notion that ethical values are an expression of divine commandment. The challenge, for today's secular society, is to make a sustainable argument for universal values which do not rely on religious precepts. Significantly, can there be a universal shared morality, notwithstanding cultural differences? Singer suggests:

[E]thics is not a meaningless series of different things to different people in different times and places. Rather, against a background of historically and culturally diverse approaches to the question of how we ought to live, the degree of convergence is striking. Human nature has its constraints and there are only a limited number of ways in which human beings can live together and flourish.[7]

This is clearly relevant for therapies which are grounded in one philosophical tradition, for example, Traditional Chinese Medicine (TCM), Ayurveda, Navajo healing, but practised in countries in which the laws and professional codes of ethics are based on another philosophical tradition. It might be the case that the ethics of health care are based on similar principles notwithstanding cultural and philosophical traditions. Singer continues:

[W]hat is recognized as a virtue in one society or religious tradition is very likely to be recognized as a virtue in others.[8]

Thus, as the role and scope of ethical theories and codes of ethics is explored, it is worth bearing in mind that even if we were to reject the applicability of western ethics to non-western CAM therapies and substitute, say, Vedic or Bhuddist ethical tradition, we would not come up with a widely divergent account of what characteristics an ethical practitioner ought to display and how ethical practitioners ought to behave. Notions of benefiting and not harming, treating patients with dignity and respect and conducting oneself with decorum can be found in all ancient texts outlining the responsibilities of physicians.

One of the earliest Chinese medical ethics texts is that of Sun Szu-miao (AD 581–682). It bears striking similarities to modern ethical codes, emphasising both professional obligations to help and the virtuous character required of a physician. The principles, summarised by Tsai, emphasise both professional obligations and virtuous character.[9]

The purpose of medical practice:

1 The object is to help, not to gain material goods.
2 Save life and do not kill any living creature.
3 Do not seek fame: virtuous conduct will be rewarded by humans and spirits.

The requirements of a great physician:

4 Master the foundations of medicine thoroughly, work energetically and unceasingly.
5 Be mentally calm and firm in disposition; do not give way to selfish wishes and desire.
6 Commit oneself with great compassion to save every living creature.

Manner of medical practice:

7 Possess a clear mind and maintain a dignified appearance.
8 Do not be talkative, engage in provocative speech, or make fun of others.
9 Do no ponder upon self-interest and fortune; sympathise and help wholeheartedly.
10 Examine and diagnose carefully, prescribe accurately and cure effectively.

Attitude towards patients:

11 Treat everyone on an equal basis, no matter whether they are rich or poor.
12 Do not reject or despise a patient who suffers from abominable diseases such as ulcers and diarrhoea: be compassionate and sympathetic.
13 Do not enjoy oneself in a patient's house while the patient is suffering.

Attitude towards other physicians:

14 Do not belittle another physician in order to exalt one's own virtue.
15 Do not discuss others and decide about their rights and wrongs.

This code, and Chinese codes of ethics following it, are underpinned by Confucian philosophy, which believes that an individual's moral cultivation is the key to achieving social order and human flourishing. Virtues such as humaneness, compassion, sincerity, trustfulness and selflessness appear repeatedly. The principles contained in these codes parallel the requirements in contemporary codes of ethics.

Re-examining the plausibility of ethical theories against the backdrop of twentieth-century atrocities, Glover argues that despite the fading of belief in a moral law, people possess certain 'moral resources' which encourage morality to prevail. His empirical observations conclude that certain human needs and psychological tendencies work against narrowly selfish behaviour. Two human responses act as a restraint in causing harm to others:

> One is the tendency to respond to people with certain kinds of respect. This may be bound up with ideas about their dignity or about their having a certain status, either as members of our own community or just as fellow human beings. The second human response is sympathy: caring about the miseries and the happiness of others, and perhaps feeling a degree of identification with them.

The second moral resource is one's moral identity, in Glover's words: 'the way we care about being one sort of person rather than another'. Healers are likely to see themselves, or wish to be seen by others, for example, as people who can be trusted, people who put the needs of their patient's before their own needs, people who keep promises and people who can be relied upon. A sense of one's moral identity, when combined with the human responses of respect and sympathy, acts as a barrier to unethical conduct. Glover notes:

> Despite the popularity of theories proposing a single basis for morality, self-interest and the different moral resources all have a role to play. Together they help to explain why, in most societies, scepticism about the moral law has not resulted in unlimited conflict and social breakdown.[10]

At the heart of CAM ethics is a universal ideal that the purpose of the healing encounter is to benefit the patient. There may be many ways in which this is done. In the current political climate of the west, it is currently thought that the best way to benefit patients is to respect their autonomy and give them the choice over their treatment. Yet, this view is relatively recent and marks a radical departure from benevolent paternalism, which, until thirty years ago, was similarly considered to be good clinical practice. This is important because many CAM practitioners work with patients who do not want to be in control and are happy for their practitioner to treat them paternalistically. Patient-centred practice would surely demand that these patients be entitled to relinquish their autonomy within acceptable boundaries. Provided practitioners are of exemplary character and are motivated by the same good intention – to benefit patients and alleviate suffering – there may be considerable latitude as to the best way to go about this. There may be competing ways of benefiting patients all of which are morally justifiable. The following chapter will explore some of the various ethical theories used in bioethics as a basis for making moral judgements.

Notes

1 Cassidy, C.M. (1996) 'Cultural Context of Complementary and Alternative Medicine Systems'. In Micozzi, M. (ed.) *Fundamentals of Complementary and Alternative Medicine*. Churchill Livingstone: Edinburgh.
2 See Kale, R. (1995) 'South Africa's Health: Traditional Healers in South Africa: A Parallel Health Care System'. *British Medical Journal*. 310: 1182–1185.
3 In the UK case of *Re T*, the Court of Appeal affirmed the right of a mentally competent adult to refuse treatment, provided the treatment refusal was valid. *Re T* (Adult: Refusal of Medical Treatment) [1992] 4 All ER 649.
4 Wong, D. (1991) 'Relativism'. In Singer, P. (ed.) *A Companion to Ethics*. Blackwell: Oxford.
5 For an overview of communitarianism, see Beauchamp, T.L. and Childress, J.F. (1994) *Principles of Biomedical Ethics* (4th edition). Oxford University Press: New York: 77–85.
6 Wong, op. cit.
7 Singer, P. (1991) 'Afterword'. In Singer, P., op. cit.
8 Ibid., pp 543–544.
9 Tsai, D. (1999) 'Ancient Chinese Medical Ethics and the Four Principles of Biomedical Ethics'. *Journal of Medical Ethics*. 25: 315–321.
10 Glover, J. (2000) *Humanity. A Moral History of the Twentieth Century*. Yale University Press: New Haven, CT.

3

ETHICAL THEORIES IN
HEALTH CARE

LIBRARY, UNIVERSITY OF CHESTER

When people are trying to decide what the right thing to do is in any given situation, they intuitively appeal to one or more ethical theories to justify their actions. An otherwise truthful person may decide to tell a lie in order to spare a patient's feelings. Another therapist may decide to disclose confidential patient information to a third party because they believe that they have a right to know. A different practitioner might keep that information secret whatever the consequences, because she has promised not to tell and thinks that people should stick to their promises. In ethical terms, these actions can be analysed as examples of consequence-based, duty-based or virtue-based reasoning. Each of these is a *normative* theory of ethics which attempts to devise a framework to distinguish right from wrong. Normative ethical theories assume that there is a criterion for knowing right from wrong, whether the criterion is a single rule or a set of rules.

The mere existence of ethical theories provides no guarantee that people will act ethically. Nor does any single theory provide a satisfactory, overarching account of what is required to lead a morally good life. It should not surprise us that ethical concepts devised in Ancient Greece or post-Enlightenment Europe offer an incomplete picture of how to lead a moral life in the twenty-first century. Newer theories have been developed, and existing theories are continually refined, to take account of current ideas about what constitutes a morally good life, espousing concepts such as non-discrimination, equal opportunity, gender equality, respect for human dignity and respect for the environment.

This chapter will present a brief overview of the ethical theories most commonly applied to health care ethics.

Consequence-based theories

Consequentialists (sometimes known as outcome-based theorists) believe that expected consequences are the main consideration in deciding whether a proposed action is ethically right or wrong. Broadly, this means that an action is right if it is expected to do more good than harm. Where it is not

45

possible to bring about a wholly good outcome, a consequential theorist would opt for the course of action which caused the least harm. This can be illustrated by returning to the earlier example of the chiropractor who knows from past experience that if she explains to a patient what a high velocity thrust feels like before she does it, the patient is likely to become tense and stiffen up, so she acts first and explains later.

In this case, the decision to withhold the information appears to undermine the patient's autonomy, but is ethically justified because the chiropractor, on the basis of her experience, knows that the consequences of providing this information in advance will be more harmful than beneficial. Since the aim of the consultation is to help the patient, the chiropractor weighs up the pros and cons and decides to deliver the intervention.

An obvious problem with a theory which makes an action ethical or unethical on the basis of the consequences of the action is that it is not always possible to know in advance what the outcome of an action will be. An action the moral agent thinks may have a good outcome, for example, a decision to withhold bad news from a patient, may have much worse ramifications than the agent might have appreciated. Rather than being grateful for being spared bad news, the patient may find out through other means and the previous relationship of trust with the therapist may be irrevocably damaged.

In order to base decisions on their likely outcomes, practitioners, as moral agents must have sufficiently strong reasons to think that certain consequences will follow. The chiropractor would only be justified in her decision if other patients had tensed up if they were anticipating a painful intervention, and the chiropractor thinks that this particular patient would react similarly. Practitioners who base decisions on the likely outcome are drawing on their practical experience and professional wisdom to help them make calculated choices. This is not the same as a decision based on gut instinct; rather, it involves reflecting on past experiences to be able to weigh up the likely positive and negative outcomes.

A second problem with consequence-based theory is that it can lead practitioners to make decisions which conflict with their patient's interests. In weighing up the pros and cons of an action, it may be necessary to take into account the effects of one's actions on third parties.

A herbalist who is attempting to control a patient's epilepsy feels morally obliged to inform the licensing authority that her patient is continuing to drive, because she believes that her patient is putting the lives of others at risk. Attempts to persuade the patient to stop driving have been unsuccessful.

Nonetheless, consequences continue to be an important component of moral decision-making, since people generally try to make decisions which will increase the overall sum of happiness for those whom their decisions affect.

Duty-based theories

Duty-based ethics (sometimes known as rule-based ethics or deontology) relies on the view that morality requires people to comply with certain duties or obligations, such as a duty not to inflict gratuitous pain on others or a duty not to lie. Duty-based approaches have much appeal in health care, since the Hippocratic tradition is rooted in the practitioner's duty to heal the sick. Proponents of duty-based theories argue that the criterion for judging whether an action is morally right or wrong is whether it follows certain rules of conduct. To duty-based theorists, the consequences of the action are not relevant and an action can therefore be moral even if it has bad consequences. Gillon observes:

> Certainly, most human societies rely in part at least on moral rules that make no reference to consequences, and it is widely accepted by psychologists that our moral reasoning is based at least in part on obedience to non-consequentialist moral rules instilled in childhood. The great religions expect obedience to moral rules (for example the Ten Commandments) that make no reference to consequences ... [1]

In addition to the moral duties of everyday life, health care practitioners, be they chiropractors or colour therapists, have additional duties towards patients which are borne out of the relationship of trust. These duties include: a duty to respect the patient's autonomy, a duty to tell the truth, a duty to maintain confidentiality, a duty to benefit patients, a duty not to harm patients, a duty to treat all patients fairly and justly, and a duty to be compassionate.

Occasionally, these duties may come into conflict. In choosing to disclose a diagnosis of bone cancer to a patient, an osteopath may cause her patient considerable distress. Assuming that the osteopath is not overstepping her professional competence in discussing the ramifications of this with her patient, it may seem like the practitioner is in breach of the duty not to cause harm to patients. The osteopath decides that her ethical duty to respect the patient's autonomy compels her to tell the truth regardless. The practitioner may be basing the decision on consequentialist reasoning. The osteopath may also be drawing on previous experience that even if breaking bad news upsets the patient initially, patients do better in the longer term if they are given help in coping with bad news and in adapting to their circumstances as best they can.

Practitioners also have to reconcile conflicting duties towards different patients.

> *A counsellor has four clients booked for one afternoon. Her first client of the afternoon has received some bad news and is very distraught. The counsellor is torn between spending more time with this client until the client is more stable or keeping the session to the usual fifty-five minutes. She feels torn between her duty to benefit the first client by giving her some extra time and her duty to benefit her other patients, who also need her. If she spends extra time with one client, she will have to spend slightly less time with her other clients, which will be unfair to them.*

This example shows that whilst duties to the individual are important, practitioners cannot devote all of their energies towards one patient to the detriment of other patients. Practitioners also need to be aware of their duties towards society as a whole, which may mean overriding their duties towards individuals. The duty of therapists to disclose details of patients suffering from notifiable diseases is another example of where duty to the individual has to yield to duty to safeguard public health.[2]

Questioning the legitimacy of rules

A problem for duty-based theories is that people are increasingly unprepared to accept rules uncritically. If this theory demands obedience to rules, therapists can reasonably ask what legitimacy the rules have and why they should obey these rules. Many duty-based theories claim to derive their legitimacy from divine law. For many centuries, people accepted the existence of a moral law uncritically. However, the collapse of the authority of religion and decline in belief in God makes philosophers and non-philosophers alike sceptical that a moral law exists or that it has a claim on us. Moreover, as Gillon points out, divine law is an inadequate justification for moral action because:

> if God were to command cruelty or injustice or wanton destruction they would be obliged to accept that these were right and morally obligatory.[3]

Other theories are derived from natural law, which maintains that some things are self-evidently right. Although divine law and natural law have an appealing simplicity as a basis for moral action, neither can provide a *universal* basis for following rules in modern secular societies.

Most rules that practitioners are asked to accept are contained in their code of ethics. The reasons for complying with the rules contained in their codes of ethics are essentially pragmatic. The first reason is that the consequences of non-compliance may include disciplinary action being taken against the practitioner. The second reason is that codes, in broad terms, represent agreement between society and professionals as to how professionals ought to act. Codes change as society changes. As patients' rights have become more visible, so codes have changed to include provisions to respect patients' values, to respect their dignity, to respect their confidences and to respect their treatment choices. In becoming a member of a professional association, a practitioner is implicitly agreeing to uphold the ethos of the professional group and to be bound by its rules. If practitioners do not comply with the standards expected of them, and professional associations do not use their disciplinary mechanisms to uphold these duties, public confidence in professionals will be lost. Accordingly, there is also a longer term economic imperative to obey the rules which govern one's profession.

For CAM therapists, the sources of professional duties vary. Within health care ethics, legitimate sources of duty include the law, professional rules and codes of ethics. Before exploring the content of these additional sources of rules, a brief account will be given on the main duty-based schools of thought which are invoked in bioethical debate.

Kantian deontology

The most influential duty-based theorist was the German philosopher, Immanuel Kant (1724–1804). Much of health care ethics is based on Kantian deontology. For the reasons outlined above, Kant argued that any theory of morality had to be justifiable without recourse to God's will, and that morality had to derive from law that humans impose on themselves. Accordingly, he devised a moral theory (his 'categorical imperative') which, he insisted, was of universal application and which any rational human being would recognise himself to be bound by.

Kantian deontologists believe that we have an obligation to act in a certain way in a given situation and that we should act in that way in every similar situation, regardless of time, place or person. If it is right to maintain confidentiality, then confidentiality must always be maintained, in every situation, regardless of the outcome. A Kantian may consider an action to be the morally right or obligatory one even if it does not promote the greatest possible balance of good over harm. Additionally, Kant argued that people should not be used as a means to an end, as this undermines their individual autonomy. This maxim would prohibit a therapist from suggesting that the patient has a few more sessions which may not be strictly necessary, simply because the therapist has received his tax bill! Most therapists would consider that they do not use patients in this way, but of course there are more subtle, if equally unethical, ways of using the patient as a means to an end, for example, prolonging the therapy because it is satisfying the practitioner's emotional needs.

The appeal of Kant to health care ethicists is the centrality his theory appears to place on respect for autonomy. Since Kant views rationality as the reason for people acting morally, it follows that respect for autonomy is ethically desirable, since it is autonomy which enables us to choose which course of action to take.

A major criticism of duty-based ethics is that the rules of conduct which are generally espoused, including respect for autonomy and a duty to benefit others, are too rigid and may conflict or lead to bad consequences. In concentrating on duty, rather than outcome, a Kantian could approve an action as morally right even if it had disastrous consequences which could be prevented. A psychotherapist may respect patient confidentiality even in the knowledge that the patient is a sex offender who is considering re-offending. A Kantian would say that confidentiality must be offered in all circumstances because it is an important facet of respecting the patient's autonomy and right to privacy, and that you cannot respect some patients' confidences but not those of other patients. A Kantian would argue that the psychotherapist should not breach confidentiality even if a patient admitted that s/he was going to perpetrate an offence. A consequentialist, in contrast, would argue that in order to maximise welfare or to prevent harm, it would be necessary and ethically justifiable to breach that patient's confidentiality, even if it meant breaking a promise to the patient to respect confidences.

Modern duty-based theories

More recent deontologists have attempted to address these criticisms whilst retaining a commitment to duty. The deontologist W.D. Ross argued that duties are a part of the fundamental nature of the universe. Certain duties are self-evident upon reflection. These include duties of fidelity, justice, beneficence and non-maleficence; all duties which are thought to be important to health care professionals. Ross also attempted to reconcile conflicting duties by introducing the idea that duties are only the first thing to consider (sometimes referred to as *prima facie* duties) and should yield to a more important duty if the situation demands it. Within Ross's duty-based theory, the psychotherapist might well feel justified in breaching client confidentiality if he thought by doing so he might avert a serious harm to an identified individual.

Rights-based theories are another version of duty-based theory. If someone has a right to something, it implies that someone else has a corresponding duty. Rights are thought to be something which we all inherently possess, such as a right to life or a right to liberty. These fundamental rights are supposedly self-evident. These rights are inalienable, that is to say, they cannot be given to somebody else. They are equal, in the sense that they apply to all humans, regardless of race, age, gender, etc. They are universal, to the extent that they apply across borders and government boundaries. The emergence of rights discourse in health care mirrors the appeal to rights in other areas (such as human rights, racial equality and queer politics). Some argue that a rights-based approach to health care ethics is an inevitable response to previous rights abuses in health care, most strikingly in the areas of medical research and mental health.

The development of rights-based theories is not universally welcomed, as some feel that it increases patients' expectations to an unreasonable degree. Many practitioners think that it is unhelpful to describe patients as consumers who have rights as this overlooks their vulnerability and need to trust, which undermines the therapeutic relationship. A criticism of rights-based arguments (a right to health care, or a right to reproduce, for example) is that they are meaningless and empty unless there is a corresponding duty to fulfil them, and in a climate of resource allocation not all rights can be met. Such arguments also overlook the extent to which rights imply responsibilities – including patient self-responsibility.

Virtue ethics

In addition to outcome-based theory and duty-based theory, a third ethical theory commonly invoked in the bioethics literature is virtue theory (sometimes known as character ethics). Although this is given less prominence than outcome-based and duty-based theories, virtue-based ethics is the oldest normative theory and is currently the subject of renewed interest.[4] Most closely associated with the ancient Greek philosopher, Aristotle, virtue theory proposes that morality is found in the development of good character traits, or virtues. This agent-centred theory states that a person is good if he has virtues and lacks vices. The virtues which are commonly invoked include benevolence, justice, prudence, fortitude and truthfulness. Additional virtues include generosity, kindness and being considerate. Within Aristotelian virtue theory, a virtue falls between two vices. Thus the virtue of courage lies between the vice of rashness on the one hand, and the vice of cowardice on the other. A moral agent must base his or her actions between the two.

Virtue theory is concerned less with the rightness or wrongness of specific actions, and more with the morality of the agent. The theory depends on the possession of virtues which will motivate the moral agent in the direction of doing the right thing. A virtuous health care practitioner will be disposed say, towards treating her patients benevolently because she knows this is the right thing to do, not because a rule imposes a sanction for not doing so. It follows that practitioners should avoid acquiring vices, such as vanity or cowardice, since this will dispose them towards acting unethically. Acting virtuously does not mean that conflicts disappear. A practitioner weighing up whether to respect a patient's autonomy or breach confidentiality will be in a difficult situation whatever the course of action taken. Even a virtuous practitioner cannot always avoid bad outcomes. Provided, however, the practitioner's action is motivated by virtue, the bad outcome does not make the practitioner a bad person.

Strong moral education is a key feature of virtue theory, because virtues are character traits which are instilled, often in youth. Consideration of virtues is particularly relevant to the training and practice of traditional therapists. Virtues do not develop overnight; practitioners become virtuous over time by performing virtuous acts until acting virtuously becomes a habit. The sort of experience required to become a virtuous practitioner may take longer than the three or four years it takes to complete a degree or a diploma in CAM and will be enhanced by emulating virtuous role models. Qi Gong masters, for example, may have received instruction from the age of 10 or even younger, often having been born into a family of traditional healers. Techniques such as herbal medicine, massage and acupressure may also have been included in this training, with ancient wisdom being passed on from master to apprentice. Moral aspects of training are an integral part of the apprenticeship.

A persisting criticism of virtue-based ethics is that virtues themselves do not lead to moral actions unless they are tied to duties to act virtuously. The virtue of veracity, for example, is unlikely to impact on the professional relationship unless the practitioner has a duty to respect autonomy and to tell the truth. Nonetheless, rules may be a useful starting point for making a practitioner do what, over the course of time, they will begin to do out of habit. Another criticism is that in focussing on a person's longer term moral character and disposition, virtue theory may overlook one-off, 'out-of-character' aberrations, such as a previously virtuous massage therapist who sexually abuses a client. The potential for therapists to cause patients harm is so great that it highlights the need to retain duty-based ethics in which specific acts are prohibited outright.

This does not mean that virtue theory has no place in CAM ethics, particularly since it concentrates on what it means to be an ethical practitioner. Rather, virtues help practitioners to refine general rules found in both duty-based and outcome-based ethics, by resolving dilemmas with an enhanced sensitivity towards the particulars of the case.

Principle-based ethics

Although it does not purport to be an entire ethical theory, principle-based ethics is widely used in the teaching of applied health care ethics. Drawing on existing ethical theories, principle-based ethics identifies four key ethical principles which appear to matter morally and which should be included in the moral reckoning whichever the theory subscribed to. Principle-based ethics is attributed to the American bioethicists, Beauchamp and Childress, and has been widely adopted by US and UK bioethicists as a tool to guide practical decision-making.[5] The four *prima facie* principles are:

- respect for autonomy
- a duty of beneficence
- a duty of non-maleficence
- respect for justice

Respect for autonomy

The principle of respect for autonomy requires the practitioner to respect the right of patients to make their own decisions in accordance with their own values. Autonomy literally means self-rule, as opposed to being ruled by others. Autonomous choosers are those who are competent and able to make rational choices; making voluntary decisions on the basis of adequate information. The assumption is that mentally competent adults are able to make up their own minds about what they do or do not want and that their views should be respected provided their views do not compromise the autonomy of others. Respect for autonomy is enshrined in patients' codes and charters.

The principle of beneficence

This ethical principle is about benefiting patients. The duty to benefit is associated with traditions of curing, helping and healing. Practitioners must be suitably competent if they hope to benefit patients, since a practitioner who does not have the requisite skills is unlikely to benefit a patient, and may also cause the patient harm. It is commonly accepted that in order to benefit, it is sometimes necessary to subject the patient to risks, but, as a rule, anticipated risks must be justified by the anticipated benefit. This implies that CAM therapists must be suitably trained and must know the risks involved in their therapy. In conventional bioethics the duty of beneficence usually refers to benefiting the patient in a physical sense. Because CAM therapists are more likely to take an interest in the patient's emotional and spiritual well-being, their duty to benefit may be substantially broader than orthodox practitioners and is likely to require a wider range of skills and competencies.

The duty of beneficence also requires practitioners to know when they are out of their depth and to recognise the limitations of their competence. The beneficent practitioner will not prolong therapy which is not having a beneficial effect, but will equally be sufficiently skilled not to terminate the therapy prematurely. The duty of beneficence also requires having the skill to know when no active intervention is the appropriate course of action.

The principle of non-maleficence

This principle requires practitioners to refrain from any behaviour which will cause the patient harm. Although it is often seen as the reverse side of the duty to benefit, the duty not to cause harm additionally implies avoidance of deliberate action which will be detrimental to the patient. Overriding the patient's autonomy, for example, by totally disregarding their express wishes, would constitute harming them. Emotional, physical, verbal or sexual abuse would certainly constitute harm. As with the duty to benefit patients, the fact that practitioners may be working on an emotional and spiritual level means that practitioners who are malevolent or insufficiently skilled may cause psychological harm or spiritual malaise to a patient. Although the law is incapable of responding to such harm, the effect on patients may be extremely damaging.

Because the outcome of any treatment can never be predicted with certainty, some would argue that the principle of not harming the patient should be seen as the primary ethical obligation, hence the medical requirement: *primum non nocere*, translated 'As the first (or primary) concern, do no harm'. One implication that this may have for CAM usage is that patients should be given the least harmful intervention first. Featherstone and Forsyth suggest:

> This means, in many cases, that complementary modalities should be applied first with the technology of orthodox medicine being used as a back up when needed.[6]

The severity of the patient's condition will also determine which option is pursued first. Chemotherapy may have more drastic side effects than following a dietary regime such as the Gersen Method, but its use as first line therapy is perceived to be justified by its likelihood of success. The problem in less acute situations, where CAM really could provide a gentler alternative, is that doctors, when they are discussing treatment alternatives with their patients, rarely provide information about options falling outside their own biomedical paradigm.

The duty of non-maleficence also requires practitioners to refrain from treating when their abilities are impaired. The British Association for Counselling require that counsellors should not counsel when their function is impaired due to personal or emotional difficulties, illness, disability, alcohol, drugs, or for any other reason.[7]

Respect for justice

This principle imposes a duty on therapists to act fairly and justly to all their clients. This implies notions of equality and non-discrimination. One aspect of justice is distributive justice, which imposes a duty on practitioners to distribute benefits and burdens in a fair and even manner. This means that therapists should allocate their time and energies equally between patients (recognising that some cases will require more intensive input at certain times than others).

The ethical principle of respect for justice denotes the need for professionals to act fairly at all times. This includes the more formalised notion of legal justice, in the form of the judiciary or the activities of disciplinary mechanisms. Legal justice implies acknowledgement and compensation when something has gone wrong. This ethical principle seeks to ensure that when harm arises, there will be fair and adequate recompense. It also requires practitioners to respond in a fair and even-handed manner to any complaints made against them.

Applying the principles

Rather than being seen as absolutes, the principles are generally understood to be *prima facie* binding. That is to say, they will apply in the first instance unless there is a good reason for them not to apply. Problems arise, however, when the principles conflict, as they so often do in real life situations. In such cases, there is no obvious pointer as to which *prima facie* duty should prevail. Although some ethicists have attempted to make credible suggestions as to how principles ought to be ranked in such situations, this remains a major problem for practitioners trying to use this approach to determine how they should act. Consider the following dilemma:

> *A healer, in a general practitioner's surgery, has been treating an elderly patient once a fortnight for three months. The patient, who is 74 and recently widowed, has rheumatoid arthritis. Although she tries to maintain her independence as best she can, the patient's mobility has become severely restricted and she is heavily dependent on others for help with her daily needs. Although the healing sessions are improving mobility, the healer is increasingly worried about the patient's depressed mental state.*
>
> *During one session, the healer notices with concern that the patient looks dishevelled and seems to have lost some weight. Although the patient is reluctant to talk, she eventually confesses that since her husband died a year ago she has lost the will to live. She says that she can't be bothered to eat and that she feels that she would be a lot less bother to everyone if she died. The healer asks if she can contact the*

*patient's GP to see about getting her some more home help. The
patient is adamant that she does not want the practitioner to interfere.*
   *When the patient misses her next appointment, the healer is thrown
into a real quandary and contemplates talking to the patient's GP,
even though her patient has specifically asked her not to.*

It is far from clear how the therapist should act. It might be useful to
consider the various ethical paths the therapist might take. In this case, the
therapist faces conflicting duties about whether to respect her patient's
autonomy and to continue to provide some limited benefit through her
healing, or whether to disregard the patient's wishes and to speak to her
GP. It is clear that the therapist is motivated entirely out of a desire to
benefit the patient and feels that the GP may be able to provide more
support than she can offer in her limited time with the patient. Nonetheless,
if she goes against the patient's wishes, she knows that she may lose her
trust and ruin the capacity for any benefit that the healing sessions may be
providing. She is concerned that to expressly override her patient's wishes
may even amount to a maleficent act, which would cause the patient more
harm than good.
   An important line of inquiry is to establish whether the patient is capable
of rational decision-making. Although the healer's training has only
included a fairly basic component on mental health, she may conclude that
the patient is suffering from depression. She may even believe that the
severity of her depression is such that the patient is non-autonomous and
that her refusal of additional assistance is a manifestation of her depression.
Without realising it, the practitioner may hold the ageist assumption that a
74-year-old patient is less likely to be as rational as a younger person and
that this is a further argument in support of overriding her wishes.
   If the practitioner genuinely feels that the patient lacks mental capacity,
she would not only be entitled, but would be duty-bound, to take such steps
as she felt to be in her patient's best interests. This begs the question of
whether the practitioner is in a position to judge this patient's mental
capacity or whether this is a matter which can only be ascertained by a
psychiatrist. Although the healer prides herself on being extremely intuitive,
she acknowledges that she has not known the patient for very long. She
accepts that she is perhaps not well placed to judge whether this patient's
refusal of assistance is consistent with her personal values or a sign that she
is 'not herself'.
   The practitioner, at this point, is likely to invoke an outcome-based
approach to justify talking to the GP. In so doing, she may be trying to
satisfy herself that this will bring about more good than harm. She may feel
confident that if the patient can be given additional help from social
services, this will decrease her sense of being a burden on her friends and
family and improve her mental outlook. She may also hope that the GP,

who has treated the patient and her husband for many years, will be able to persuade her to take better care of herself. Yet, it is far from certain that the practitioner's intervention will result in the desired outcome. It may be that, as a result, the patient becomes the subject of scrutiny and is judged to be incapable of looking after herself and is coerced into going into a home, thus losing the last vestiges of her independence. If the practitioner is going to base her decision on future consequences, she must have a strong reason for thinking that her intervention will be beneficial not harmful.

Alternatively, the practitioner may decide that she is more motivated by duty than consequences and that her duty to respect the patient's wishes not to talk to the GP outweighs any possible consequences of doing so against the patient's wishes. As a patient-centred practitioner, the healer may choose to accept the patient's wishes and recognise that in terms of her own assessment of her quality of life, the patient may have legitimate reason for feeling that she is a burden on her carers and that without her husband, she would rather die. Again, it would be important for the practitioner to reach a decision as to whether the patient was indeed autonomous, since her duty would shift from one of respect for autonomy to a duty to act in her best interests if the patient were not competent.

The practitioner may also be motivated by other factors, including her concept of herself as someone who keeps her word, and for this reason, she may choose to respect her implied promise not to intervene. As a practitioner committed to acting compassionately, she may consider trying to achieve the same ends by providing the patient with information about self-help groups and bereavement counselling, thus empowering the patient to seek further assistance should she so desire.

This case study demonstrates that it is not always obvious how a practitioner ought to act and that there may be more than one ethically justifiable approach. Ultimately, decisions will need to be based on the facts of the individual case and no formulaic guidance can determine which principles should take precedence in the particular instance. The main problem with abstract principles is they cannot embrace the uniqueness of the individual case. Jonsen and Toulmin argue:

> The heart of moral experience does not lie in a mastery of general rules and theoretical principles, however sound and well reasoned those principles may appear. It is located, rather, in the wisdom that comes from seeing how the ideas behind those rules work out in the course of people's lives: in particular, seeing more exactly what is involved in insisting on (or waiving) this or that rule in one or another set of circumstances. Only experience of this kind will give individual agents the kind of practical priorities they need in

weighing moral considerations of different kinds and resolving conflicts between those considerations.[8]

Another significant criticism of the principles approach is that it assumes a shared morality in which principles such as respect for autonomy are highly valued. This may be the case in the USA and the UK, but this does not mean that each of the principles is equally valued in other cultures. As in the above case, therapists should be aware of their own values and biases since these may cloud their professional judgement.

Nonetheless, the principle-based approach is a widely used teaching tool in bioethics, and each of the four principles is an important area of moral concern. The principles cannot of themselves, however, reflect the range of values upon which ethical health care practice is predicated, and for this reason we must now look beyond ethical theory and consider other approaches to determining the morally right course of action to pursue.

Notes

1   Gillon, R. (1986) *Philosophical Medical Ethics*. John Wiley & Sons: Chichester.
2   In the UK, the Public Health Act 1984 imposes a statutory duty on doctors to notify local authorities about a list of notifiable diseases. Many CAM codes of ethics extend this duty to inform practitioners.
3   Gillon, op. cit, 15.
4   For a good summary, see Crisp, R. (1996) 'Modern Moral Philosophy and the Virtues'. In Crisp, R. (ed.) *How Should One Live? Essays on the Virtues*. Oxford University Press: New York.
5   Beauchamp, T.L. and Childress, J.F. (1994) *Principles of Biomedical Ethics* (4th edition). Oxford University Press: New York.
6   Featherstone, C. and Forsyth, L. (1997). *Medical Marriage: The New Partnership Between Orthodox and Complementary Medicine*. Findhorn Press: Findhorn, Scotland.
7   British Association for Counselling (1990) *Code of Ethics and Practice for Counsellors*. British Association for Counselling: Rugby.
8   Jonsen, A.R. and Toulmin, T.S. (1988) *The Abuse of Casuistry: A History of Moral Reasoning*. University of California Press: Berkeley, CA. Cited in Murray, T. (1997) 'What Do We Mean By "narrative ethics"?'. In Lindemann Nelson, H. (ed.) *Stories and their Limits. Narrative Approaches to Bioethics*. Routledge: London and New York.

4

PROFESSIONAL CODES
OF ETHICS

The second important source of ethical guidance for consideration are professional codes of ethics. Codes of ethics are seen as an integral part of patient protection because they establish the ethical standards expected of the practitioner and provide a benchmark against which a practitioner can be held accountable. Yet, the extent to which these influence practitioners' behaviour is questionable, given that not all practitioners belong to a professional body and not all professional bodies maintain an up-to-date code of ethics reflecting current practice. Because some therapies have become professionalised only relatively recently, there has been a tendency for professional bodies to borrow a code of ethics from elsewhere (often another therapy) and to apply it uncritically to their practitioners. Other professional bodies have a code of ethics, but do not have corresponding disciplinary mechanisms to enforce its standards, so that adherence to its provisions is arbitrary.

Assuming that it would be possible to devise a more appropriate code of ethics, would this provide an effective source of practical guidance? Many would argue that if therapists are professional, they should be acting ethically in any event. If therapists are not minded to act ethically, then arguably, a code of ethics which lists a range of 'Thou Shall Nots' is not going to turn them into model practitioners. It may be dispiriting to think that codes of ethics should have to rely on their deterrent effect, but practitioners do take the notion of accountability more seriously if they think their practice is likely to be judged against the provisions of the code and that breaches could potentially lead to disciplinary mechanisms. This may be even more necessary in CAM, where other regulatory controls, such as litigation or employment tribunals, are lacking.

Before evaluating how far professional codes of ethics can influence behaviour, it is necessary to consider what is meant by the term 'professional' and whether it can be assumed that true 'professionals' are disposed towards acting ethically.

What is a professional?

Since the 1990s, many CAM therapies have striven towards greater professionalisation. For many therapies this has meant the willingness to work alongside therapists who have a slightly different orientation to their own, the merging of overlapping professional registers and the creation of accreditation processes designed to ensure consistent training requirements. Most therapists consider this to be a good thing, even if they themselves have little interest in taking an active part in the politics of their profession. Any therapist who has undergone a rigorous training will not want to work alongside therapists who have had only minimal training, because if harm is caused to patients this reflects badly on the group as a whole.

Moves towards professionalisation imply a more rigorous approach to policing the profession. High training standards and effective disciplinary mechanisms are seen as central to protecting patients from harm. Some therapists think that professionalisation will enhance their own status. The more professional the therapy, the more highly the individual practitioner will be regarded. However, there are a lot of misconceptions about the nature of professionalisation and the advantages and disadvantages of different types of regulation.

What expectations are created by describing a relationship as 'professional'? A lay person would probably describe a professional relationship as a business-like arrangement, with services provided by someone who knows what they are doing. When a sick person consults a health professional he wants to know that the practitioner is someone who can be trusted to act in his interests, who will treat him with courtesy and respect as an individual and, above all, who is skilled at what he does. To be thought of as a professional is to be considered safe and trustworthy.

But who decides when an occupational group merits the privilege of being accorded 'professional' status, and on what basis? Increasingly, almost every occupation claims (or aspires to) professional status. It is not unusual to hear the words 'professional hairdresser' or 'professional football player'. Whilst both occupations require a high level of technical skill, what they lack, in comparison to professional health care practice, is a lengthy training, systems of accountability and a commitment to ethical practice and serving the public interest. Because the term 'health profession' implies a high level of competence and trustworthiness, governments are unlikely to award therapies the status of statutory regulation unless they have already demonstrated high levels of effective voluntary self-regulation.

What is a profession?

Cant and Sharma list membership of a professional association, a codified knowledge base and altruistic values as being some of the traits common to professionals.[1] These are thought to explain the high status and authority of professionals. However, they postulate that more recently, professions have been described in relation to the strategies they have utilised to attain their positions of status, authority and monopoly provision. Such strategies include social closure, state support, market control and technical authority. Specialised knowledge (characteristically acquired through a long and formal academic route) is also seen as central, since this both legitimates high status and promotes social closure, by restricting use of that knowledge to those few who have acquired this knowledge. This may explain why nursing is not viewed as having the same professional status as medicine. Although nursing has an increasingly technical knowledge base, the more routine and caring aspects of nursing are thought to be tasks which anyone (particularly women) can perform. It may provide a partial explanation for why certain CAM therapies, such as healing, are portrayed more as vocations than professions.

Do professions serve the public interest or self-interest?

Despite this supposed commitment to public service, a key question is whether professional groups are predominantly motivated by public interest or self-interest. Are some CAM therapists motivated by status and prestige more than a desire to benefit patients? Although both desires may operate concurrently, this issue tends to be looked at in binary terms, rather than accepting that a stronger professional base can benefit both patients and practitioners. Ogus[2] describes two rival conceptual models of the origins of regulation which he terms the 'public interest' and the 'public choice' models. The 'public interest' approach explains regulation as a mechanism by which economic and social activity is controlled in the interest of what is perceived to be the good of society. The contrasting 'public choice' approach broadly represents regulation as a commodity which is obtained from the governing and administrative establishment by competing interest groups within society who wish to secure regulation in order to protect their own interests.

This is relevant for the present debate because numerous commentators have described the history of conventional medicine as the ultimate example of protectionism through which doctors have not only been able to secure a monopoly of health care provision, but have also established themselves as the ultimate arbiters of what constitutes health and health care. Certainly, the rise of conventional medicine in the nineteenth century saw a relative decline in the fortunes of alternative healers whose right to practise was taken away or heavily circumscribed.

Despite agitation by the medical profession to introduce clauses into the UK's 1858 Medical Act to restrict practice to those medically qualified, the Act did not give the medical profession a full monopoly. It did make it illegal for unqualified practitioners to describe themselves as being medically qualified. The Medical Act ensured that thereafter, the state would employ registered medical practitioners. Since the training of registered medical practitioners excluded unorthodox practices, and early General Medical Council (GMC) professional codes forbade association between doctors and non-conventional practitioners, alternative medicine was effectively marginalised. By aligning themselves with the dominant scientific paradigm, doctors managed to secure a professional base in which their authority was assured and their professional accountability rarely called into question. It is only relatively recently that the GMC has bowed to public pressure and begun to revise its regulatory structures.

If it is felt that professional regulation for the medical profession made doctors more concerned with their own status and power, it is curious why so many CAM practitioners view the pursuit of professionalisation as desirable. The same fundamental tension between public interest and professional self-interest also operates within CAM regulation. In the UK, where osteopathy and chiropractic are currently the only two statutorily regulated CAM therapies, other therapies are actively pursuing statutory regulation. A desire to raise standards is clearly one reason to pursue statutory regulation, but the anticipation of greater status and reward is another. Protecting the profession from conventionally trained practitioners is another reason to define one's group as a profession.

Behaving ethically: individual and collective responsibilities

The decision whether or not to behave in an ethical manner is ultimately a matter for the individual practitioner. Ethics, it has wryly been said, is what practitioners do when nobody else is looking. Most CAM encounters are characterised by private practitioners seeing patients alone in their own home, or in a closed room in a clinic. No-one can look over the shoulder of a practitioner the whole time and there is ample scope and opportunity for unethical practitioners to abuse their patients' trust. An argument against training practitioners about ethics is that if someone is intent on acting unethically, they will do so in any event. This book is not just concerned with avoiding the worst examples of practice, but promoting the optimum standards of care. For this reason, it is necessary to look not just at the individual therapist's responsibilities, but at those of the profession as a whole. Stacey describes the difference as follows:

> Individual therapeutic responsibility is exercised by the practitioner in the encounter with a client or patient. Collective therapeutic responsibility is expressed in the formal rules or advice promulgated by organizations of practitioners which guide or restrain individual practitioners in encounters with patients or clients. The purpose of such rules or guidance is to control the standards of practice and

behaviour of members. When those formal rules or guidance have statutory backing the constraints experienced by the practitioner are tighter because the sanctions which the professional body may exercise have legal authority.[3]

Certainly, all practitioners must be accountable for their own actions. Hopefully, most therapeutic encounters are ethical and the patient has no reason to be dissatisfied. Most anxieties and concerns will hopefully be able to be addressed at the level of individual practitioner and client. But some aspects of ethical practice can only be co-ordinated at a collective level if they are to provide protection to patients as a whole. The responsibilities of professional bodies include:

- determining educational requirements for safe and competent practice at pre- and post-registration levels;
- encouraging research and professional development;
- setting standards through codes of ethics and codes of practice;
- maintaining and making available a register of members so that the public can determine regulated practitioners from unregulated practitioners;
- maintaining professional disciplinary procedures so that unethical practitioners can be held accountable for their actions;
- having a complaints mechanism whereby patients may have their grievances heard and any appropriate reparation made;
- putting in place mechanisms for dealing with practitioners unfit to practise through ill health;
- providing information to members of the profession;
- providing information to members of the public and promoting patient self-awareness.

Professional bodies are an integral aspect of ensuring ethical practice. If, however, the ethical responsibilities of the professional bodies are going to have any impact on the behaviour of practitioners, other than in a top-down, authoritarian sense, a third set of obligations needs to be considered, namely, the duties of individual practitioners to participate in, and share responsibility for, collective professional structures.

Most therapists are willing to take responsibility for their own ethical propriety, but do not see themselves as having any direct responsibilities towards collective aspects of professional responsibility. Practitioners value their professional autonomy and tend to harbour hostile thoughts towards their disciplinary body, which they may regard as hostile or interfering. This is regrettable, bearing in mind disciplinary bodies are there to perform the critical task of protecting the public. It is also ethically damaging, since it casts the regulatory body and, indeed, the regulatory process as *external to the practitioner*. Unless practitioners feel that they 'own' their regulatory body, they will have less regard for the rules it sets. If practitioners have not contributed to collective standard setting, they will seek to bend the rules, determining that the rules might be appropriate for other people, but which don't take account of the way in which they are special and therefore exempt from their scope.

Being a professional confers rights and responsibilities. The right to self-regulate is a significant privilege which should not be underestimated. It is an acknowledgement of a government's trust that the *profession as a whole* is capable of setting high standards of practice and conduct, will respond to public grievances and will contribute to education and research. In the case of CAM, failure to exercise that responsibility could result in the right to self-govern being taken away and replaced with direct government control.

Taking this argument further, a profession is made up of individual practitioners. Each therapist has a responsibility to make these things happen. *Professional regulation is not someone else's responsibility*. It is the composite responsibility, exercisable jointly and severally, of each individual member. This responsibility is analogous to the legal concept of a partnership, where each partner is responsible for the actions of other partners. This is not a new idea. Almost every professional code of ethics exhorts members to protect and promote the good name of the profession. Yet, individual practitioners assume that this professional requirement does not extend to them, or that if it does apply, it certainly doesn't require any positive duty on the practitioner's part. This view is misguided. Promoting the name of the profession does involve individual responsibility, over and above refraining from poor practice in one's own practice.

As with any true partnership, this change of culture will require commitment from both individual practitioners and professional bodies. Responsibilities on the part of individual practitioners to promote the common good might include some or all of the following:

- willingness to make suggestions as to how ethical codes could be made more relevant to practice;
- willingness to serve on preliminary investigating and professional misconduct committees;
- willingness to participate in profession-wide peer review schemes;
- willingness to act as a supervisor or mentor to newly graduating practitioners;
- willingness to participate in research trials;
- willingness to respond to consultation exercises on policy initiatives.

Corresponding action will be required on the part of professional regulatory bodies to reduce the sense of alienation felt by members.

Professional codes of ethics as a source of ethical guidance

Ethical codes provide a number of functions. The primary function of a code of ethics is to ensure public protection by setting out the ethical requirements of practitioners. To fulfil this function, codes of ethics not only need to be in existence, but they need to be enforced. The second function is to serve as a reminder for practitioners of what their ethical responsibilities are. A third possible function is to inform patients of their rights and what they can expect from their practitioners. Many professional bodies fail to seize the public relations potential of this aspect of maintaining a code of ethics and do not routinely make their code available to members of the public, or only do so at a price. An obvious way in which professional bodies could make themselves more accessible is by posting their codes of practice on a website, since patients increasingly use the internet to help them select a practitioner.

A code of ethics cannot provide a blueprint for action. No single code could possibly hope to set out how a practitioner should behave in any conceivable situation. Rather, codes of ethics provide general statements of intent, and are usually couched in general, aspirational terms which take little account of the specific context of the therapeutic encounter. Although most professional associations vaunt the mere existence of a code of ethics as some kind of guarantee of ethical practice, closer reflection might reveal that these codes, albeit of important symbolic value, have little effect on how practitioners actually work or upon the quality of ethical decisions they make.

The scope of ethical codes

A code of ethics represents the ethos of any given profession. Health care is a moral enterprise in which health carers are dedicated to the welfare of their patients. This involves putting their patients first, causing no harm, and using their skills to benefit those who need them. Surprisingly, although these codes are intended to encourage ethical practice, they rarely make explicit the ethical foundations upon which they are based. A newly qualified practitioner may be given a list of prohibitions, but it is not clear from the text why these rules ought to be followed, or why the code prioritises certain issues over others. In fact, most codes combine duty-based ethics and virtue-based ethics. Most codes draw heavily on the principles of respect for autonomy, beneficence and non-maleficence, and also stress the character requirements (or virtues) of an ethical practitioner.

Codes of ethics can be seen as a synthesis of minimal legal requirements and statements of ethical ideals, backed up with professional statements which represent the shared political and economic ideals of that particular group. Within medicine, a central problem in devising ethical codes has been that the goal of healing the sick has occupied an uneasy position alongside the promotion of self-interest. Pellegrino and Relman assert that:

For centuries, a commitment to the effacement of self-interest has been embedded in traditional codes of medical ethics but has never been actualized as the vital spirit of professional organizations. Too often, ethical goals have been commingled with protection of self-interest, privilege and prerogative.[4]

In the past, codes tended to reflect professional self-interest, at the expense of the patient's interest. For example, early ethical codes considered it professional misconduct to denigrate a fellow professional. In contrast, a modern code, such as the General Osteopathic Council's Code of Practice, *Pursuing Excellence*, states that a practitioner must:

Act quickly if they believe a colleague's conduct, health or professional performance – or their own – may pose a threat to patients.

Most codes of ethics have been rewritten in recent years to take account of the shifts towards patient-centred practice and the obligations on the health practitioner to act competently and with integrity. The adoption of a code of ethics by a professional organisation, and the agreement of members to be bound by its provisions, serves as a reminder that professionals do have ethical duties over and above those of ordinary people and that their obligation to society is not merely based on economic self-interest.

To provide practitioners and patients with some practical advice, rather than statements of lofty intent as to desired character traits, the bulk of provisions flesh out some of the practical requirements associated with the commitment to respect the patient's autonomy, to benefit and not cause harm, and to respect the principle of justice.

Autonomy based requirements include:

- a duty to respect the patient's values and cultural beliefs and to make sure that personal beliefs do not prejudice patient care;
- a duty not to abuse the patient's trust;
- provisions relating to consent;
- provisions concerning the treatment of minors and mentally incapacitated adults;
- provisions relating to confidentiality, including when confidentiality may be breached.

Beneficence/non-maleficence requirements include:

- the need to maintain and develop professional skills;
- recognition of the limits of competence and when it is appropriate to refer the patient;

- a statement acknowledging the scope of professional practice, for example, whether the therapist can make a medical diagnosis;
- the need to maintain accurate, comprehensive records;
- the duty to work in an open and co-operative manner with the patient's medical practitioner and other health care professionals;
- the duty to report poorly performing practitioners to the appropriate professional body;
- a requirement that the practitioner be physically and psychologically fit;
- a requirement that the practitioner complies with relevant legal provisions;
- the need to maintain appropriate professional indemnity and professional liability insurance;
- the duty never to abuse one's professional position.

Character/virtue requirements include:

- a requirement to act with integrity and uphold the core values of the profession;
- a recognition of the fiduciary nature of the relationship.

Notably, very few CAM codes explicitly include justice requirements. Codes rarely compel practitioners to comply with the notion of distributive justice by encouraging members to make their services available to all sectors of society who wish to avail themselves of them. This is perhaps not that surprising, given that most CAM therapies operate largely in the private sector. Whilst individual practitioners may well operate a sliding scale for patients who could not otherwise afford to consult them, few professional bodies advise on this problem of equity of access as a collective issue. In response, professional bodies may consider the feasibility of lending their support to subsidising *pro bono* work amongst its members. Some organisations do already do this and include specific provisions in their code of ethics to this effect. For example, the American Chiropractors Association's Code includes this clause:

> Doctors of chiropractic should support and participate in proper activities designed to enable access to necessary chiropractic care on the part of persons unable to pay such reasonable fees.

Indeed, a criticism of most professional codes of ethics is that they do not attempt to make any reference to the political and economic realities in which their profession operates. Nor do they question the theoretical basis from which they are derived. The British Association for Counselling provides a fine exception to this, and attempts to contextualise its advice in the following extract from its revised Code:

One of the characteristics of contemporary society is the coexistence of different ways of approaching ethics. This statement reflects this ethical diversity by including values, principles and virtues that are considered essential to the talking therapies. This selection of ways of expressing ethical commitments does not seek to invalidate other approaches. However setting different ways of conceiving ethics alongside each other is intended to draw attention to the limitations of relying too heavily on any single ethical approach. Ethical principles are well suited to examining the justification for particular decisions and actions. However reliance on principles alone may detract from the importance of the practitioner's personal qualities and their ethical significance in the counselling or therapeutic relationship. Virtues direct attention to this aspect of professional ethics. The provision of culturally appropriate and sensitive services is also a fundamental ethical concern. Cultural factors are often more easily understood in terms of values.

Since ethical codes can never predict every ethical scenario which is likely to arise, and advice has to be of a general nature, the question arises: What should go into an ethical code? A balance needs to be drawn between providing minimal advice in the form of vague, generalisable statements (which nobody could take issue with, but which fail to provide any real guidance) and providing detailed advice which is overly prescriptive. As an example, most codes of ethics for acupuncturists specify: 'Patients should be provided with enough information to make an informed choice.' This allows the acupuncturist to use her discretion as to how much information this particular patient receives, and in what form. Compare this with a hypothetical advice that mandates:

> Before treating a patient you must be sure that the patient understands the broad principles of Yin and Yang theory, the Five Elements, the organ systems, and the origins of Qi.

Not only is this likely to be impractical, it is also likely to be unnecessary, and would limit the ability of the practitioner to tailor the disclosure to the needs of the individual. Professional codes also need to recognise that different members may utilise widely differing therapeutic techniques and work with a broad range of patients. A single code of ethics for psychotherapists may need to cater to Jungian, Freudian, Kleinian, humanistic and eclectic therapists, working with adults, children, adolescents, families, groups or offenders. A code of ethics can easily incorporate these differences provided the advice is limited to generalised ethical ideals, representing the core values of the profession.

Because codes provide general advice, it is the practitioner's responsibility to apply ethical rules to *the particular circumstances of the case*. Some codes in fact stress that all practitioners are accountable for their own actions and must be prepared to justify their decisions. The Code of the British Association for Counselling makes this point in its revised guidance to its membership. Its Statement of Fundamental Ethics for Counselling and Psychotherapy reads:

> This statement indicates an important change in approach within the Association. Previous codes were presented as prescriptive and thus requiring conformity by all members. The prescriptive approach has been rejected as undermining the practitioner's personal responsibilities for being ethical. It has also proved impractical to prescribe uniform practice across the diverse field of counselling and psychotherapy without fostering unethical practice by some members. Instead, a much greater emphasis is being placed on the practitioner's own responsibility to think and work ethically. This Statement draws on the collective experience of this Association in order to inform and inspire best ethical practice.

Advantages and disadvantages of professional codes

Codes of ethics are often criticised for failing to offer any practical support for practitioners who are faced with an ethical dilemma. This may be a fair criticism, particularly where the code fails to address the ethical basis upon which it claims to base its legitimacy. Other disadvantages of ethical codes are:

- codes provide general advice only so they are not helpful in specific instances;
- codes tend to be negatively couched, emphasising what practitioners must not do, rather than how they ought to behave;
- unless codes are kept regularly up to date they may give misleading advice, especially on practitioners' legal requirements;
- codes are often drafted without consumer input, even though a major part of their function is to protect consumers;
- codes are drafted with insufficient input from membership, and thus might be out of touch with day-to-day problems arising in practice.

But professional codes of ethics cannot be taken in isolation from the other regulatory functions of professional bodies. Arguably, the function of professional bodies in setting high, uniform *educational* standards has a more direct impact on whether practitioners will go on to practise ethically. The existence of effective grievance procedure sends a strong message out to consumers that the professional body takes its responsibilities to the public very seriously and that unethical practitioners will be dealt with severely. This confidence can, of course, be lost, if the actuality of professional disciplinary mechanisms is that practitioners are hardly ever disciplined, or are allowed to carry on practising even after they have been found to guilty of serious professional misconduct.

Since most ethical practitioners would regard their code of ethics as offering little by way of practical guidance, and do not seem to guide action, is there any particular reason for professional bodies to continue to provide codes of ethics? Since professional bodies continue to disseminate codes of ethics, and governments when they are considering therapies for statutory regulation insist that members work to a code of ethics, it is presumably thought that ethical codes do, on balance, contribute towards ensuring high ethical standards. Advantages of ethical codes include the following:

- codes give practitioners a framework within which to work – this can be particularly helpful for therapists who work alone in private practice and do not have regular contact with other practitioners, and for the vast majority of therapists who do not take an active role or interest in the politics of their profession
- codes proscribe certain specific forms of activity, and in doing so, provide disciplinary procedures and courts with a basis for determining whether a practitioner's conduct was acceptable
- codes give patients an idea of what sort of conduct they can reasonably expect and demand from practitioners
- by setting down core values of conduct expected of practitioners, codes ensure consistency of ethical behaviour amongst practitioners on the same professional register who may work in a variety of different contexts, quite possibly utilising very different therapeutic methods

The existence of a professional code of ethics is only one aspect of a larger strategy that professional bodies must adopt to foster high ethical standards within its profession. Indeed, the failure of existing statutory health care bodies to protect the public is a clear indication that promoting ethical practice requires more than lip service on the part of professional associations. In the future, public pressure may force regulatory bodies to abandon their top down, hierarchical approach, in favour of a collective approach to self-governance in which individual practitioners assume shared responsibility for the standards and development of their profession.

Notes

1   Cant, S. and Sharma, U. (eds) (1996) *Complementary and Alternative Medicines. Knowledge in Practice*. Free Association Books Ltd: London.

2   Ogus, A.I. (1992) 'Regulatory Law: Some Lessons from the Past'. *Legal Studies*. 1: 4.
3   Stacey, M. (1994) 'Collective Therapeutic Responsibility. Lessons From the GMC'. In Budd, S. and Sharma, U. (eds) (1994) *The Healing Bond*. Routledge: London and New York.
4   Pellegrino, E. and Relman, A. (1999) 'Professional Medical Association. Ethical and Practical Guidelines'. *JAMA*. 282(10), September 8.

5

THE LAW

Therapists must work in accordance with the law and be familiar with any particular legal rules which affect their sphere of practice. There is a large degree of similarity between what is ethical and what is legal. Since morality and the law are often derived from the same Judaeo-Christian sources, one would expect this to be the case. An important difference between ethics and law is that ethical guidance aims to promote optimal standards of conduct. Determining what is ethical involves weighing up competing rights and considerations to arrive at the best outcome in the circumstances – or the least bad option, if all choices are problematic. The legal duty of care requires only that therapists act as a 'reasonable practitioner' would act in similar circumstances. If the common standard within a therapy is high, then the patient will be afforded a higher level of protection, but if standards within a profession are generally low, then the standard required of a reasonable practitioner will be correspondingly sub-optimal, and patients will not be very well protected.

The legal relationship between CAM practitioners and patients is contractual. This means that the practitioner and patient have entered into a voluntary agreement, whereby the practitioner will provide professional services in return for appropriate compensation (usually in the form of fees for service). Unlike business contracts, which are usually in writing, most contracts with patients are verbal. Practitioners are not *obliged* to enter into a contract with any particular person. An aromatherapist may legitimately decide that she only wants to work with female clients. A sports therapist may decide he only wishes to take on professional athletes as clients. Legally, a practitioner cannot be forced to work with particular clients or groups of clients. Sexual and racial discrimination legislation largely excludes private practitioner/client relationships. Ethically, one expects practitioners to treat all prospective patients in an even-handed and non-discriminatory fashion. If a practitioner feels that he is unable to take on a particular client, he should do what is possible to ensure that person is able to access appropriate help from someone else.

What is the legal duty of care?

As with ethical responsibilities, all therapists owe their patients a duty of care. A therapist is under a legal duty to act with the *due care and skill* of a responsible practitioner. This implies that a therapist will be able to help and will not harm a patient, that the practitioner will respect the patient's rights, for example, to privacy and confidentiality, and that the practitioner will deal with the patient in a fair and non-discriminatory way.[1] Since few therapies are capable of causing a patient serious, lasting side effects, until now there has been very little litigation against CAM therapists. Whether this will change as therapists become more professionalised and achieve a higher status and income remains to be seen.

Currently, it is difficult to sue a therapist if their therapy lacks professional standards or if the therapist is unaffiliated to a professional group and uninsured. Even in the USA, where litigation against health care practitioners is rife, most patients would not dream of accessing formal law as a means of redress, even if they had been seriously harmed by a CAM practitioner, so the absence of litigation is not necessarily indicative of an absence of poor practice.

The main reason for highlighting the lack of litigation against CAM therapists is that the absence of legal redress makes it all the more important that practitioners act ethically and professionally. The penalties imposed for breaking the law may be taken more seriously by therapists than the moral opprobrium for acting unethically. Certainly, criminal law penalties are an effective deterrent, since they can ultimately result in loss of liberty. However, the impact of acting unethically on both the individual patient and the professional as a whole should not be underestimated. If practitioners abuse the professional relationship, they may find that their freedom to practise is significantly curtailed.

Criminal law

All practitioners are subject to the criminal law. Whereas negligence involves unintentional acts, to be found guilty of a crime, a person must have both committed the unlawful act and intended to have done so. Few practitioners exhibit the criminal intent necessary for a court to establish that a crime has been committed. Because health care relationships involve a high degree of trust, courts deal very severely with practitioners who commit offences against their patients. Most professional bodies regard a serious criminal conviction either as automatic evidence of serious professional misconduct, or as a basis to initiate disciplinary proceedings, whether or not the prosecution is related to professional activities. If a practitioner is minded to commit a criminal offence, it is unlikely that a series of prohibitions contained in a code of ethics will serve as much of a deterrent. Practitioners who suspect other practitioners of unlawful activity should report this to the relevant professional body in order to protect patients from harm.

Civil law

Law suits between practitioners and their patients are more likely to be brought under civil law. Civil law is the branch of law which deals with disputes between individuals. In most jurisdictions, the legal actions most likely to be brought against a therapist are in trespass (otherwise known as assault or battery), which protects the patient from unwanted touching, or in negligence, for failure to treat the patient in accordance with professional standards.

Trespass

A patient who sues for trespass does not have to show that she was harmed, merely that the practitioner interfered with her bodily freedom. A practitioner might be liable of trespass for:

- touching a patient without any consent whatsoever;
- failing to provide even a basic explanation of what is going to be done to the patient;
- lying to the patient about what will be done, so that any consent which has been given is vitiated by fraud or misrepresentation;
- going beyond that for which consent had been obtained.

Trespass, then, is the legal action which most closely protects a patient's autonomy from unwanted interference. Examples of potential trespass might include an osteopath who performs an intimate examination without express consent, a chiropractor performing a risky procedure without giving the patient any information about potential risks, or a massage therapist gaining consent to perform a massage, but then doing something different and unexpected, such as inserting some acupuncture needles. In each situation, the patient is likely to have agreed to undergo treatment, but has not given their express permission for what took place. Actions in trespass against health practitioners are uncommon but not unprecedented.

Negligence

Practitioners working in increasingly litigious societies are more likely to be concerned about being sued for negligence. Many practitioners think that any professional mistake may result in a negligence action. This is not the case. Practitioners will only be held liable for mistakes which are negligent, that is, mistakes which fall below the standard expected of a reasonable practitioner. Significantly, negligence involves *unintended* mistakes, unlike criminal acts, which require the prosecution to prove criminal intent as well as criminal action. The difference in moral terms is significant, because we think that it is right to hold people to account for their deliberate actions, on the basis that they ought to know the difference between right and wrong. Unless a practitioner is grossly negligent, harm which a practitioner causes to a patient through an unintentional mistake does not confer the same implication of culpability that a criminal allegation does. Consider the following:

> *A naturopath at a residential spa is using a combination of hot and cold bath treatments to improve a patient's circulation. Unfortunately, the thermostat has been altered without the practitioner's knowledge and the water temperature is hotter than she intended it to be. She fails to check the temperature of the water by hand, and the patient is scalded. Her client is distraught, but forgiving.*
>
> *Later the same day, the naturopath is treating a patient who has been extremely abusive to her and the other practitioners at the spa. She deliberately fills the bath with scalding water and protests that she did not realise the thermostat had been changed. This client is outraged and calls the police.*

In an action for negligence, the burden of proof is on the patient to prove, on a balance or probabilities,

* that the practitioner owed the patient a duty of care;
* that the practitioner was in breach of that duty; and
* that the breach of duty caused the patient harm.

A practitioner can be negligent by act or omission. A practitioner can be liable for acting in breach of one's duty of care, or by failing to act when a reasonable practitioner would have acted. In CAM, it may be easier for a patient to establish a negligent omission than commission. A medical herbalist who prescribed a combined remedy which included a blood thinning substance might be negligent if she failed to take a full history and did not discover that the patient was simultaneously taking conventional blood thinning medication, as a result of which the patient suffered blood loss from a severe cut. By contrast, it may be uniquely difficult to establish what a reasonable practitioner would have done, particularly in a CAM practitioner therapy for which there are no agreed standards or competencies, or where opinion is sharply divided. This point will be taken up in the next section.

Miscellaneous legal requirements

CAM practitioners are also subject to a raft of miscellaneous provisions, often affecting the business side of their practice. These may impact on ethical practice, by demanding standards of conduct and safety which improve the general welfare of patients. Various local licensing provisions may apply to practice premises and use of equipment. Property and tenancy agreements may make certain stipulations about seeing clients from home, and practitioners should ensure that if they see patients from their own home that they are not in breach of a restrictive covenant which prohibits the use of residential premises for business purposes. Therapists who set up a practice at home must be adequately insured for any harm which may be occasioned to patients on their premises. If the therapist is not the owner of the property, the landlord should be informed before the premises are used for business purposes. Since it is important to provide continuity for clients, practitioners should take legal advice concerning any premises they intend to use for consultations. Particular thought should be given to premises which are shared by a number of practitioners.

> *A homoeopath sees patients at a group practice. Whilst she is on maternity leave, she enters into an agreement with a locum, who takes over care of her patients for her at the same location. Unfortunately, as the locum is showing an elderly patient from the waiting room to the consulting room, he trips on some loose carpet and breaks his ankle. He sues the practice for damages for personal injuries. The homoeopath has signed a written agreement with the other practitioners agreeing that they be jointly responsible for maintenance and structural repairs. Although she is on maternity leave at the time of the incident, the homoeopath is liable for her share of the damages as specified by the legally binding agreement.*

Various statutory provisions also affect aspects of CAM, including health and safety legislation, data protection legislation, and regulations governing the claims which can be made about treatments and medicinal products. Compliance with these provisions is ethically necessary since they are designed to protect consumers from harm and respect patients' rights. It is the practitioner's responsibility to ensure that they are aware of, and comply with, any relevant legal provisions.[2]

Shortcomings of law as a means of regulation

The law serves as an additional regulatory control over practitioners whether they are statutorily regulated, voluntarily self-regulated, or working in an entirely unaffiliated manner. Nonetheless, legal controls operate retrospectively, and particularly in the case of criminal and civil law, are only likely to be invoked once a patient has already been harmed. As a preventative strategy, the law does little to prevent patients from harm or to raise standards within a profession generally.

As a means of regulation, legal mechanisms are unduly formalistic, burdensome and prohibitively costly, making them inaccessible to the vast majority of CAM patients. Moreover, the lack of litigation against CAM practitioners means that judges have little awareness of CAM relationships and have few tools for analysing an adverse incident or deciding how responsibility should be allocated. Whilst the law determines minimal standards of conduct, it has little use in promoting the high standards of conduct desirable in any CAM relationship.

Notes

1   As well as this common law duty, private CAM practitioners also have a statutory duty towards their clients under the Sale of Goods and Services Act 1982.
2   For further discussion of legal aspects of CAM practice, see Cohen, M. (1998) *Complementary and Alternative Medicine: Legal Boundaries and Regulatory Perspectives*. Johns Hopkins University Press: Baltimore, MD and London, Dimond, B. (1998) *The Legal Aspects of Complementary Therapy Practice*. Churchill Livingstone: Edinburgh, and Stone, J. and Matthews, J. (1996) *Complementary Medicine and the Law*. Oxford University Press: New York.

6

DO ALTERNATIVE THERAPIES REQUIRE AN ALTERNATIVE ETHICAL FRAMEWORK?

The question should now be raised whether the sources of guidance discussed previously provide an adequate basis to guide moral action? The question assumes that ethical decisions are based, at least in part, on ethical theory. This, in itself, is a contentious proposition. There is little empirical evidence as to how far clinicians draw on ethical theory in arriving at (hopefully) ethically defensible positions, or, indeed, how far anyone relies on overarching theories in determining right from wrong. Some philosophers argue that our grasp on moral traditions and theories is so patchy and incomplete that theory alone cannot provide an adequate basis for action.

Recourse to theory may not provide a wholly convincing justification for moral action. Psychological and political factors will also influence how a practitioner acts.

A student osteopath has become very attached to an elderly client, who reminds the student of her late grandmother. The student tries to arrange this patient's appointments at the end of a session, so that she can spend more time with her than other clients. An audit of the clinic shows that this student sees fewer clients than other students and spends more time with them than has been allocated. Since the unit is hoping to attract NHS funding, the clinic directors cut appointment times from forty minutes to thirty minutes, so that the clinic can increase throughput. The student responds to this by spending a few minutes less with her other clients so that she can continue to provide 'special' treatment to her elderly client. She knows that this is unfair to her other clients, and is even jeopardising her end-of-year results, but feels that this client has come to rely on her and has no-one else to talk to.

CAM practitioners, as moral agents, will be motivated to act in certain ways for a variety of reasons which may appear compelling in one situation and not in another. Few practitioners, one suspects, feel that they need a thorough understanding of moral philosophy before they take a client's history. Yet, as moral agents engaged in the pursuit of improving health and relieving suffering, therapists must reflect on why they make the decisions they make, and how they can build on this knowledge to make better decisions in the future. The therapeutic relationship, of its very nature, puts the therapist in a position of considerable power and influence. In order to use that power responsibly and to the benefit of patients, practitioners need to develop greater ethical awareness, and to build critical reflection into their professional practice.

In terms of individual ethical decision-making, two of the three sources of ethical guidance already discussed, namely professional codes of ethics and the law, are largely non-negotiable. Anyone choosing to practise *must* comply with the laws of the country in which they are practising. Similarly, if practitioners belong to a professional body, they must comply with its professional standards, or else face disciplinary action. There is undoubtedly scope for refining the laws which apply to professional practice and improving professional codes, making them more relevant to the nuances of CAM practice. Nevertheless, practitioners are obliged to work within the law and the standards set by their professional body.

This means that if a legal requirement is at odds with a practitioner's cultural norms, the law of the land will prevail. An example of this is the Anglo-American requirement to gain informed consent before providing treatment. This legalistic approach to the therapeutic relationship may be at odds with a practitioner's values or cultural or philosophical background. Many CAM therapies, for example, originate from cultures where paternalism is more highly valued than individual autonomy. *This does not provide the therapist with licence to avoid consent requirements.* Similarly, if a code of practice requires the practitioner to be honest with their patients at all times, a practitioner cannot argue that in his culture it is felt better to withhold bad news and preserve the patient's hope. At the same time, both law-makers and professional organisations are morally bound to consider cross-cultural implications and how these can be most fairly reflected.

Can we apply western values to non-western therapies?

The question to raise is can we apply western values to non-western therapies? Do the ethical theories which have been considered provide an adequate basis for thinking about ethical decision-making in CAM, or are they too rooted in western philosophical tradition to be of much interest to non-western practitioners?

Many CAM therapies are rooted in western healing traditions. However, many indigenous and ancient healing traditions draw on profoundly different cultural belief systems and traditions. Within the ethical literature there has been little systematic attempt to ask whether it is appropriate to apply western values and ethical traditions to therapeutic traditions derived from non-western systems. Failure to address this question may lead to cultural misunderstanding and the imposition on practitioners of ethical obligations which are at odds with their traditional forms of practice. Eskinazi notes:

> Traditional health care systems represent philosophical approaches to managing health and disease that differ substantially from those of Western biomedicine. The question of what is common to these traditional systems has been largely overlooked, but spirituality is an integral part of each. As this trait is often directly related to the dominant religion or philosophical system of the originating culture, it is taken for granted within the context of health care. For example, the ancient Chinese health care system was influenced by several spiritual schools, in particular Taoism. Ayurveda, a traditional medical system of India, reflects the traditional Hindu world view. Similarly, Tibetan physicians practice Buddhist meditation as an integral part of their medical training.[1]

Nowhere are the fundamental and irreconcilable differences more stark than between philosophies underpinning western scientism and eastern mysticism. An area in which this is most manifest is that a background in science is not a necessary precondition for training in many CAM therapies. Some people come to practise therapies directly out of an interest in eastern religions and philosophy. Unlike medical students, they simply do not come to training or practice with a scientific, empirical mindset. They may profoundly reject intellectualism and rationalism in favour of a more intuitive approach. If this is true for a proportion of therapists, it is probably also true for a proportion of the patients who consult them. Realistically, it may be inappropriate to insist that these therapies adduce scientific proof that their therapy works, since the practitioners may have neither the interest nor the skills to carry out formalised health care research. Forcing these practitioners into an evidence-based, empirical mindset would be fundamentally at odds with their values and philosophies about the universe, and those of their patients.

Yet, despite the huge diversity of healing traditions across the world, they all share the same underlying goal of relieving suffering, promoting health and protecting the health of the wider community. Cassidy explains that systems arise because they serve a need, and that patients report satisfaction with care if it is delivered in a manner which coincides with their cultural expectations of a healing encounter. She makes the important point that:

The form health care takes is first and fundamentally a matter of sociocultural interpretation. In other words, the 'truth' that guides any health care system is relative and is learned.[2]

In China, patients routinely receive traditional treatment in a large room in front of other patients. A history is likely to be taken with no privacy, no curtain and no soundproofing.[3] A non-Chinese patient would almost certainly regard this as an unwarranted breach of her privacy and as a deliberate undermining of her autonomy. How much does it matter if the therapist and the client have a different cultural background or understanding of how a therapy works? Discussing Chinese medicine, Ergil argues:

> Culture is a complex network of signification, elements of which might resonate only in a very local sense while other aspects have almost global relevance. This does not mean that the medical ideas and practices of one society cannot and will not be successfully appropriated by another, but rather that aspects of a system that are meaningful to one group of people may not be meaningful at all to another.[4]

What issues arise when healing customs and practices are divorced from their traditional underpinnings and re-packaged for a western market? Acupuncture provided by doctors in a UK or US hospital-based pain relief clinic may achieve some benefit, but this may not compare to the successes which can be achieved when acupuncture is delivered to patients who are culturally cognisant with the notion of 'Qi' (vital energy) and can describe accurately the point at which the needle has 'obtained the Qi' (known as *de Qi*). Based on his experiences as the first US medical exchange student to study Traditional Chinese Medicine in China, Eisenberg comments:

> Most Chinese have experienced acupuncture. They are not unduly frightened by it and they understand the phenomenon of *de Qi*. In fact, the patient guides the acupuncturist by saying when an acupuncture needle has hit its mark and elicited the appropriate sensation. By contrast, most Western patients seeking acupuncture know nothing of the phenomenon of *de Qi*. Not knowing what sensations they should anticipate, they cannot tell the acupuncturist when a needle is in the right place. When both the therapist and patient know little about *de Qi*, as frequently occurs in Western acupuncture clinics, the result is bound to be disappointing.[5]

If we accept Cassidy's point that all belief systems are relative and that what matters is that the healing system coincides with the patient's belief system, some of the potency of traditional practices is likely to be lost when they are used in a westernised setting. This is an important question which gives rise to hitherto unasked ethical questions. With reference to understanding health systems in their cultural perspective, Ergil points out:

> It is easy to make intellectual errors when dealing with medical systems. We forget that our own perspectives may prevent us from understanding the meaning and utility of practices that have been developed within another culture. That failure to account for our own needs and biases can lead to the overenthusiastic acceptance of ideas whose genesis and application we do not really understand.[6]

Many patients commit enthusiastically to alternative systems of health care even if they do not understand or embrace the underlying philosophy on which the therapy is based. Patients do not seem to need to understand how a therapy works in order to receive some benefit.

Are traditional therapists selling out in some way if they adapt their therapy to make it more culturally acceptable? Taking a medical history in China, for example, a Traditional Chinese doctor may ask the patient a list of directive 'yes' or 'no' questions. That same doctor, if treating private patients in the UK or USA, is more likely to ask patients open-ended questions which allow the patient to explore how they feel and make patients feel like they are having their voice heard.[7] One could argue that when practitioners decide to work within a dominant culture, they recognise that their patients will be influenced by this and may alter their practice accordingly, or they may not. These are unsettling questions but ones which have profound implications for the integration of non-western therapies and indigenous healing practices with conventional medicine.

Since all health care practice is predicated on the same ethical ideals of relieving suffering and not causing harm, CAM may not require an entirely new ethical framework. What the above discussion reveals, however, is that there may be grounds for reviewing ethical theories and considering how these might be supplemented by other theoretical standpoints which are better able to accommodate therapies which do not fit within the dominant paradigm scientifically, politically or philosophically.

Alternative ethical theories

Traditional bioethics has tended to adopt a Kantian framework which supports modernist, reductionist approaches to health care, characteristic of allopathic, conventional medicine. Nowhere is this more obvious than Kantian deontology, and in its focus on universality, rationality and autonomy. As Hekman observes:

Kant defined an entity that has become the centerpiece of modern moral theory: the disembodied subject, a subject that knows no culture, history, class, race or gender.... Furthermore, the laws that this autonomous subject legislates and executes (the political terms here are no accident) are moral only in that they are universalizable; the deciding factor in moral judgments cannot be particular circumstances, concrete empirical conditions, but must be the universalizability of the abstract principle. That women are excluded from this realm should be obvious but, just in case his readers have missed the point, Kant notes: 'of course, I exclude women, children and idiots.'[8]

It is little wonder that CAM therapists may have picked up conventional bioethics textbooks and thought that this subject has little to offer them or their practice. What is needed is a broader range of ethical theories which recognises and builds on the shortcomings of existing theoretical models. CAM requires ethical theories which are sensitive to its broader philosophical underpinnings, and are appropriate for therapies which favour a therapeutic approach which values individual differences as well as universalisable similarities, intuition in addition to rationality, and dependence as well as autonomy.

But even if therapists find the ethical tools previously discussed unhelpful or inadequate, they are deeply rooted in western consciousness. Most of us base moral decisions partly in accordance with rules and perceived duties, partly in anticipation of the likely outcome, and partly based on the sort of person we would like to be thought of by others. Therapists also make decisions about their patients in this way, whether they consciously acknowledge it or not.

Two ethical theories may be helpful to this discussion, namely: care-based ethics and narrative-based ethics. These theories are not intended to replace those already discussed, but to supplement them in order to provide a fuller account of what it means to act ethically.

Ethics of care

Feminist theory is concerned with the extent to which women's perspectives have been largely discounted from the dominant fields of human inquiry, not least of all in the fundamental area of knowing, in which the male-dominated view is highly sceptical of subjective, intuitive forms of knowing, favouring instead rational, objectivity. The ramifications of this are significant, given the link between knowledge and power. As Bowden observes:

The exclusion or devaluation of the significance of caring relations by philosophers, political theorists, historians, social scientists,

economists, lawyers and physicians, imposes a dominating understanding of knowledge that masks its exploitation of those relations
and the oppression of the (mostly female) persons whose lives are
shaped by the obligations of care.[9]

This exclusion has significant repercussions for how we view the ethics of
CAM medicine. Sexual politics continue to be a significant issue in health
care. Nursing politics has pushed for a greater recognition of the healing
potential of the more personal, 'human', touch-based skills of nursing. This
has coincided with a considerable interest among nurses in many of the
complementary and alternative therapies. This can be seen as a desire to
shift the balance away from the impersonal, mechanistic style of much
modern medicine towards the more personal, nurturing, gentle bias that is
characteristic of the 'feminine' approach to healing.

An ethics of care has emerged out of feminist theory. Carol Gilligan's
work has been particularly influential in this regard. She highlights the
activity of caring, the process of communication and the mutual dependence on the maintenance of relationships.[10] Autonomous individuals are
located within a web of relationships whereby:

> [r]esponsibility now includes both self and other, viewed as different
> but connected rather than as separate and opposed.[11]

Rejecting Lawrence Kohlberg's theory of moral development as failing to
take into account the fact that women's moral experience may be different
from that of men, Gilligan researched the way in which women make moral
decisions. Her research found 'empathetic connectedness' to be central to
women's moral decision-making. Whereas men, in Gilligan's terms, display a
'justice orientation', women display a 'responsibility orientation'.

Kohlberg's work, based on research on adolescent boys, viewed the moral
agent in Kantian terms, as being someone who objectively analyses moral
dilemmas using rules and principles to make rational choices.[12] Kohlberg,
like Kant, placed a high priority on individual autonomy, human rights and
personal liberty. Moral problems are seen as conflicts and solutions are
reached by ordering rights.[13] The ethical theory underpinning this approach
is impartialism, that is, 'the view that ethics is based upon impartiality,
impersonality, universal principle, and formed rationality'.[14]

Gilligan conducted her own research on women facing the moral
dilemma of whether to terminate a pregnancy. Her findings formed the basis
of her groundbreaking book: *In a Different Voice: Psychological Theory and
Women's Development*. This argued that women are not inferior in their
personal or moral development, as Kohlberg's framework suggested. There
are profound distinctions in the ways in which men and women frame and
resolve moral problems. Females typically view morality in terms of respon-

sibilities of care deriving from attachments to others, whereas males typically see morality in terms of rights and justice. Gilligan did not purport that the female mode of thinking about morality was limited to women, rather that women *tend* to affirm an ethics of care that centres on responsiveness in an interconnected network of needs, care and the prevention of harm, as men *tend* to embrace an ethic of rights suing quasi-legal terminology and impartial principles, accompanied by dispassionate balancing and conflict resolution.[15] This has obvious implications for the CAM therapeutic encounter. Here Gilligan's formulation of an alternative framework for viewing morality shows that it is possible to have competing pluralities in moral matters, rather than viewing morality within one particular (male-centred) framework.

An ethics of care provides an important counterpoint to the prevailing view that respecting individual autonomy is the foremost value in western democratic societies. Other ethical considerations, particularly caring, may be more important in the healing relationship. Caring refers to caring for, emotional commitment to, and a willingness to act on behalf of persons with whom one has a significant relationship. Within an ethics of care, Kantian universal rules, impartial utilitarian calculations and individual rights are all downplayed. What matters within an ethics of care is not simply *what* the practitioner does, but *how* she does it. An ethics of care is involved with the motives which underlie moral actions and whether moral actions promote or thwart relationships with patients.

Critically, Gilligan's work provides theoretical support for the role of dependency in the CAM relationship. Harbison comments:

> In Gilligan's vision, dependence is assumed to be part of the human condition; being dependent is not regarded as being helpless and powerless, but simply being convinced that people have an effect upon each other, and recognising that interdependence empowers both. The reference for moral judgment now becomes not oneself, but the relationship between self and others.[16]

This view of dependence may account for the willingness of some CAM patients to relinquish their need for control and to be prepared to rely and depend upon their therapists for the duration of the treatment episode. Beauchamp and Childress note that:

> [T]he desired moral response [to patient vulnerability, dependence and illness] is attached attentiveness to needs, not detached respect for rights. Feeling for and being immersed in the other person establish vital facets of the moral relationship.[17]

Further support in favour of the relevance of care-based ethics to CAM ethics can be derived from the work of Nel Noddings. Bradshaw describes Noddings's perspective as follows:

> Noddings articulates a feminine perspective on care which involves a kind of indwelling relationship, an engrossment and motivational displacement derived from feminine emotional qualities. The carer finds her true self when she chooses to become involved in caring relationships. Thus Noddings contrasts these specifically feminine caring attributes with what she perceives to be the detached, rational and analytical coolness of male thinking. She wants to emphasis the subjectivity and emotionality of caring *and the uniqueness of each caring relationship.*[18] (italics added)

Many CAM therapists would be reassured to hear a description of morality which so closely mirrors their therapeutic approach to care. An ethics of care may provide some theoretical support for the intuitive way in which CAM therapists respond to individual patients. Within an ethics of care, an appropriate and considered response to any given moral dilemma might be: 'I'm not sure. It depends on the situation and the relationship I have with that client.'

For Tronto, an ethic of care is a practice, rather than a set of rules or principles. An ethic of care has four elements: attentiveness to the needs of others; taking responsibility, having sufficient competence to provide good care; and the responsiveness of the care-receiver to the care. The need for care challenges the idea that all individuals are autonomous and self-supporting. Tronto maintains that recognising vulnerability in others, and being responsive to the needs of the vulnerable person, should alert the care-giver to the possibility of abuse arising out of vulnerability, not least of all the assumption that the care-giver can define the needs of the vulnerable.[19]

Nonetheless, care-based ethics has been criticised on a number of fronts. Allmark[20], for example, makes the point that care-based ethics assumes that caring (remembered from one's experiences of childhood), at the centre of care-based ethics, is automatically a good thing. Care, he argues, is only good when it has been *good caring*. Caring may be smothering and stifling and thwart the goals of the person being cared for. He also disputes the contention that caring is a moral quality in itself, because it depends what one cares about. Care-based ethics assume that the things that the carer cares about are morally good, whereas they could be morally neutral or morally bad. In these situations, the qualities required of the carer, in terms of sensitivity and skill to bring about the caring, may similarly be morally neutral or bad.

Narrative-based ethics

Narrative-based ethics is a theoretical approach to ethics which has been gaining increasing currency in recent years. In contrast to previously discussed ethical theories, narrative-based ethics stands out as a necessarily individualistic theory, which is well suited to patient-centred practice. The strength of a narrative-based approach is that it not only places the patient's story (narrative) at the centre of the therapeutic encounter, but that it also takes account of the highly contextualised framework in which the patient relates to his or her own experience of illness. Narrative-based ethics recognises the role that the patient's narrative forms as part of a life story.

Significantly, narrative-based ethics also takes into account the extent to which the medical encounter can distort what the patient is actually saying, and reconfigure it in a different language with a different meaning. Its attraction as an additional ethical tool is that it forces the therapist to acknowledge the unequal distribution of power in the relationship and to recognise that the therapist is making value-laden judgements when he or she privileges one narrative or interpretive framework over another. Greenhalgh and Hurwitz suggest that in the *therapeutic process*, narratives:

- encourage a holistic approach to management;
- are themselves intrinsically therapeutic or palliative;
- may suggest or precipitate additional therapeutic options.

In *research*, they argue that narratives:

- set a patient-centred agenda;
- challenge received wisdom;
- generate new hypotheses.[21]

Unlike other ethical theories, the narrative-based approach suggests that the practitioner's character and intent is not all that matters from a moral point of view and allows the moral subject to assume centre stage in their story. This might capture something of what is meant by CAM therapists when they claim to work in a patient-centred way.

For Arthur Frank, author of *The Wounded Storyteller*, narrative is central to an understanding of illness and healing. Narrative, for Frank, is the method through which patients reclaim their illness, formerly only validated through the official interpretation of medical experts. He explains:

Folks no longer go to bed and die, cared for by family members and neighbours who have a talent for healing. Folks now go to paid professionals who reinterpret their pains as symptoms, using a specialized language that is unfamiliar and overwhelming. As patients, these folks accumulate entries on medical charts which in most instances they are neither able nor allowed to read; the chart becomes the official story of the illness.... The story told by the physician becomes the one against which [other] narratives are ultimately judged true or false, useful or not.... I understand this obligation of seeking medical care as a *narrative surrender* and mark it as the central moment in modernist illness experience.

What is distinct in postmodern times is people feeling a need for a voice they can recognize as their own. This sense of need for a personal voice depends on the availability of the means – the rhetorical tools and cultural legitimacy – for expressing this voice. *Postmodern times are when the capacity for telling one's own story is reclaimed.* Modernist medicine hardly goes away; the postmodern claim to one's voice is halting, self-doubting and often inarticulate, but such claims have enough currency for illness to take on a different feel.[22]

Modernist medicine, Frank argues, claimed the body of the patient as its territory. The patient was robbed of the right to the particularity of his or her own experience of illness, suffering being reduced to medicine's general view. Research into why people use CAM reveals that patients want this individualised approach to care and to feel that they are being heard and understood.

A thirty-two-year-old woman has gone to her GP because she has been suffering from repeated stomach cramps, bloating in the evening, and more or less permanent diarrhoea. Although her GP appears to be very interested in hearing about her physical symptoms, the patient is angry that he glosses over her psychological explanation attributing her symptoms to the stress of looking after her mother, who has just undergone major heart surgery, and the difficulties she is experiencing at work from an unsympathetic manager. The GP diagnoses irritable bowel syndrome and prescribes medication. When this fails to alleviate her symptoms, she follows a friend's advice and goes to see a homoeopath. She is relieved when the homoeopath specifically asks her what she thinks is causing her symptoms and takes this into account when prescribing the best treatment. The patient finally feels that someone has taken her views into account and responds well to her individualised remedy.

Narrative is especially important to the CAM relationship if we accept that the relationship between the practitioner and client has a therapeutic value in itself. Recognising that good communication accounts, in part at least, for the efficacy of CAM encounters, Johannessen makes the point that:

The clinical conversation is an important tool in the creation of individualized explanations and treatments, and it may be a kind of individualized therapy in itself.[23]

She continues:

[I]ndividualized explanations hold great potential for meaning in treatment. When patients get individualized explanations and treatments of the often chronic ailments for which complementary medicine is sought, it is likely to create order in the personal chaos accompanying sickness. This ... creation of meaning could be significant not only for the illness experience of the patient but also for the healing processes in the patient's body and disease.

Anti-authoritarians challenge the way in which purportedly 'objective' medical knowledge is used by doctors as a basis for privileged interpretation of the patient's story. As Brody points out:

[T]he exercise of power is a social and political act, and no theory of scientific objectivity, however well grounded, automatically grants the sort of privilege that medicine has traditionally claimed for itself as a social enterprise.[24]

Although CAM therapists are less 'guilty' of favouring their interpretation over patients than perhaps doctors have been in the past, it would be facile to think that power differentials do not exist in the CAM/patient relationship and that CAM therapists do not, on occasion, use that disequilibrium in ways which are damaging to patients.

Narrative-based approaches to bioethics may offer a more patient-centred approach than other ethical theories. But as Brody continues, simply recognising the power wielded by the health professional will not make problems disappear:

As more and more people see the world in the new way, and start to see choices where the old world view saw only inevitability, then change will come, but change will not amount to the wholesale dismantling of what we call modernism. Some practices and some power relationships will persist, because there is a good reason for them to persist, or because alternative arrangements turn out to have even more problems.[25]

His sentiments may provide an interesting justification for the high levels of paternalism within CAM relationships today and why paternalism persists in CAM, even though it is discredited in orthodox medicine. If most practitioners are more concerned with making patients better than eliciting their opinions, this suggests that there is a place for dependency and reliance within the therapeutic relationship.

Narrative-based approaches to bioethics may offer a more patient-centred approach than other ethical theories. Nonetheless, it may be hard to see how a narrative-based approach really differs in practice from respecting the patient's autonomy, which, properly understood, already encompasses taking account of the patient's personal and cultural value systems. Moreover, a focus on the patient's narrative, and their right to tell their own story, overlooks the distortion and self-deception that telling one's story often entails. Patients are free to rewrite their history, and arguably, whatever story they want to tell about themselves has authenticity. However, the unreliability of the narrator deprives practitioners of the ability to base treatment decisions and make moral judgements on objective facts.[26]

A further shortfall of this approach is that holistic therapies can be patient-centred without necessarily focussing on the rational, articulated views of the patient. An intuitive CAM practitioner can 'read' the body, be it an acupuncturist reading pulses and observing the tongue, a masseur sensing areas of muscle tension, or a bioenergetics practitioner finding clues to the a patient's disease in the patient's chronic body postures. In this way, a diagnosis can be reached without even eliciting a verbal history or narrative from the patient. Indeed, the emergence of narrative-based ethics at a time when the principle of respect for autonomy is already perceived to be so important might indicate the extent to which the commitment to respecting autonomy derives from a fear of being sued, rather than from a desire to provide optimally patient-centred care.

Notes

1 Eskinazi, D. (1998) 'Factors that Shape Alternative Medicine'. *Journal of the American Medical Association*. 280(18), November 11.
2 Cassidy, C.M. (1996) 'Cultural Context of Complementary and Alternative Medicine Systems'. In Micozzi, M. (ed.) *Fundamentals of Complementary and Alternative Medicine*. Churchill Livingstone: Edinburgh.
3 Eisenberg, D. with Wright, T.L. (1995) *Encounters with Qi. Exploring Chinese Medicine*. W.W. Norton & Co., Inc.: New York.
4 Ergil, K. (1996) 'China's Traditional Medicine'. In Micozzi, M., op. cit.
5 Eisenberg, D., op. cit.
6 Ergil, K., op. cit.
7 Eisenberg, D., op. cit.
8 Hekman, S.J. (1995) *Moral Voices, Moral Selves: Carol Gilligan and Feminist Moral Theory*. Polity Press: Cambridge. Quoted in Clarkson, P. (2000) *Ethics. Working with Ethical and Moral Dilemmas in Psychotherapy*. Whurr Publishers: London.
9 Bowden, P. (1997) *Caring: Gender Sensitive Ethics*. Routledge. London and New York.
10 See Gilligan, C. (1992) *In a Different Voice: Psychological Theory and Women's Development*. Harvard University Press. Cambridge, MA.

11 Ibid., 147.
12 Kohlberg, L. (1981) *Essays in Moral Development*. Harper & Row: New York.
13 For a thorough analysis see Harbison, J. (1992) 'Gilligan: A Voice for Nursing?' *Journal of Medical Ethics*. 18: 202–205.
14 Allmark, P. (1995) 'Can There Be an Ethics of Care?' *Journal of Medical Ethics*. 21: 19–24.
15 Beauchamp, T.L. and Childress, J.F. (1994) *Principles of Biomedical Ethics* (4th edition). Oxford University Press: New York: 85–92.
16 Harbison, J., op. cit.
17 Beauchamp and Childress, op. cit.
18 Bradshaw, A. (1996) 'Yes! There Is An Ethics Of Care: An Answer For Peter Allmark'. *Journal of Medical Ethics*. 22: 8–12.
19 Tronto, J. (1993) *Moral Boundaries: A Political Argument for an Ethic of Care*. Routledge: London and New York.
20 Allmark, P., op. cit.
21 Greenhalgh, T. and Hurwitz, B. (1998) *Narrative Based Medicine: Dialogue and Discourse in Clinical Practice*. BMJ Publishing: London.
22 Frank, A. Cited in Brody, H. (1997) 'Who Gets to Tell the Story? Narrative in Postmodern Bioethics'. In Lindemann Nelson, H. (ed.) *Stories and Their Limits. Narrative Approaches to Bioethics*. Routledge; New York and London.
23 Johannessen, H. (1996) 'Individualized Knowledge: Reflexologists, Biopaths and Kinesiologists in Denmark'. In Cant, S. and Sharma, U. (eds) *Complementary and Alternative Medicines. Knowledge in Practice*. Free Association Books Ltd: London.
24 Brody, H., op. cit.
25 Ibid.
26 Arras, J. (1997) 'Nice Story, But So What? Narrative and Justification in Ethics'. In Lindemann Nelson, op. cit.

Part II

ETHICAL ISSUES COMMON TO ALL THERAPISTS

Introduction

In Part I, a strong case was made for increasing the ethical awareness of CAM practitioners. All health care practitioners, whatever their therapeutic orientation, owe their patients an ethical and legal duty of care. As well as considering relevant ethical theory as a basis for moral action, practitioners also need to work within the guidance of their professional associations and the law. No two therapies or therapists are the same, and how practitioners ultimately fulfil their ethical obligations will vary from relationship to relationship. Because external systems for ensuring accountability of CAM practitioners are of varying quality and usually only come into play when a patient has already been harmed, individual therapists must regulate their own conduct. Hopefully, a willingness towards acting ethically can be assumed. Part II of this book will explore how to put that commitment into practice.

This part of the book sets out the core ethical requirements of any therapeutic encounter. The choice of topics for discussion are divided into three themes previously identified as relevant to all healing relationships, namely: (1) benefiting patients and not causing them harm; (2) respecting patient's autonomy; and (3) acting fairly and justly in dealings with patients. Not surprisingly, these issues form the bulk of most professional codes of ethics, which, as previously discussed, draw heavily on principle-based ethics. The guidance and prohibitions contained in codes presume a shared or common morality whereby the rightness of the contents are assumed to be self-evident. Even though health carers may share a common objective of healing the sick, the content and scope of ethical duties is not self-evident and requires further exploration.

A further justification for an avowedly principle-based grouping of ethical issues is that this currently represents the dominant approach to bioethics. If there is to be constructive dialogue between CAM practitioners and conventional health care practitioners, there needs to be a shared vocabulary. Since there has been no systematic attempt within CAM to develop an ethical vocabulary of its own, CAM therapists should consider how the language of bioethics fits with their own models of health and healing.

Although the topics are presented as discrete ethical areas, in practice there is considerable blurring. It could be argued, for example, that many of the issues related to respecting a client's autonomy belong in a general discussion of benefiting and not harming. Similarly, the need for therapists to provide adequate complaints mechanisms are as much a component of the duty to benefit and not harm as they are a justice requirement. In terms of balance, it should not be a surprise that the bulk of the material in this section deals with benefiting and not harming, since these are the issues which are the major cause of ethical concern in complementary and alternative medicine. Some of the issues discussed will be more relevant to some therapies than others. Therapists are urged to reflect on the information in this section and think about how the issues raised affect their own practice. The subjects for discussion are as follows:

Issues related to benefiting and not harming

- Competence
- Research
- Supervision
- Continuing professional development
- Maintaining boundaries and preventing abuse

Issues related to respect for autonomy

- Respect for autonomy and consent
- Truth-telling
- Confidentiality and patient records
- Negotiating contracts with patients
- Duties towards children and mentally incapacitated adults

Issues related to justice

- What to do when things go wrong

7

COMPETENCE

Key ethical issues:
- What is competence and who defines it?
- How useful are formalised competencies?
- Making realistic claims
- Recognising limits of competence
- Effective collaboration with other health professionals
- Cross-specialisation
- How far can training ensure competence?

A principle ethical concern is that unless practitioners have the requisite competence to be able to benefit and not harm patients, they should not be working as health professionals. Patients consult CAM therapists in the hope and expectation that the practitioner will be able to benefit them at best and not harm them at worst. In ethical terms, these reflect the duties of beneficence and non-maleficence. A therapist who is not competent cannot hope to help or benefit a patient and may cause harm. Accordingly, determining competence is an ethical, as well as a technical, imperative.

What is meant by competence?

A fundamental principle of ethical practice is that therapists have the necessary skills to practise their particular therapy. At the most basic level this requires them to have sufficient therapeutic skills to provide safe, effective treatment. Without these skills, it is unethical for therapists to offer therapeutic services to patients. Although this sounds obvious, the diversity of training offered within any given therapy means that the amount of knowledge and practical experience that a therapist might require to obtain a qualification varies enormously. CAM practitioners may offer services after a four-year training or four weekend courses. In such a climate, it may be hard for a member of the public to know whether the therapist they consult is competent or not. Palmer Barnes defines competence as follows:

> Professional competence implies a standard of practice that in Winnicott's terms is 'good enough'.[1]

Using Winnicott's notion of 'good enough' parenting, this definition serves as a useful reminder that professional competence does not imply excellence, rather it refers to levels of good practice which other practitioners would consider reasonable. This provides the professional standard against which an individual practitioner's standards can be measured, and sets a professional benchmark against which ethical and legal duties can be measured.

Competence includes technical aspects, relationship aspects and professional practice aspects of a therapist' work. Ideally, professional training ought to provide a would-be practitioner with the requisite skills to practise their chosen therapy. As well as having the requisite skills to practise, other factors may affect competence to treat in a specific instance. A therapist may have acquired sufficient clinical experience to qualify as a practitioner, but may still feel out of his or her depth with a particularly challenging client. Competence also involves monitoring one's practice. Critical reflection is an essential part of good practice and ensures that practitioners learn from their experiences, good or bad.

What competencies are required of a CAM practitioner?

It may be extremely difficult to determine the competencies required of a CAM professional because the diversity in training standards is so great. The requirements laid down by professional associations vary significantly and many practitioners work in an entirely unaffiliated fashion. One way of considering whether a practitioner is competent is to consider whether they can meet certain competencies. There are certain core skills that all therapists should have in order to be able to practise. These key skills will be relevant no matter what therapy, or combination of therapies, the therapist is using with a patient. This is important because the harm that most patients suffer is not necessarily due to want of technical proficiency. These skills might include:

- good history-taking skills
- observational skills
- listening skills
- communication skills
- documenting skills
- ability to arrive at a differential diagnosis
- application of theoretical knowledge to clinical encounter

Failure to demonstrate these competencies may result in significant harm to the patient, as the following examples demonstrate:

Taking an incomplete history

A fifteen-year-old patient from a Hassidic Jewish family is taken to see a herbalist because of bloating and persistent stomach ache. A combination of an inadequate history taking, together with cultural stereotyping, leads the herbalist to overlook any possibility that this patient may be sexually active. In fact, she is five weeks pregnant. The herbalist prescribes thuja, which has an abortifacient effect.

Failure to diagnose

A nutritional therapist is attempting to control a patient's psoriasis. The patient also complains of being tired all the time and feeling generally unwell. An exclusion diet is recommended in which the patient is only allowed to eat nuts and bananas for a fortnight. When the patient returns, she has lost fifteen pounds and is still feeling unwell, although her psoriasis has improved slightly. The therapist introduces a slightly less restrictive regime and tells her to return in another two weeks. The patient is subsequently diagnosed as having stomach cancer.

Whether the harm in each situation could lead to legal action, as well as a disciplinary complaint, would depend on what a reasonable practitioner would have done in similar circumstances. The first example highlights the need to establish any factors which rule out a particular therapy. The second example raises the controversial question of how much medical knowledge a therapist needs to make an accurate diagnosis and to know when to refer.

Problems in formalising competencies

Who defines competence?

Ideally, the competencies required of a therapist in any given therapy should be determined on a collective level by the profession as a whole. In order to determine training and practice standards, professional groups need to set aside differences and concentrate on their commonalities. This is best done on a therapy by therapy basis. If competencies were designed in this way, then there could be agreed differences to take account of different therapeutic approaches within a given therapy, whilst ensuring basic levels of safety.

One problem with this approach is that, historically, only the most professionalised schools and associations become involved in defining competencies. Although politically active, these bodies may not be representative of the therapy as a whole. The more alternative and less politically affiliated groupings may have profoundly different ideas about what competencies their profession requires, but their relative disenfranchisement means that their views will not be incorporated. Accordingly, competencies and other professional matters will be decided by the most mainstream groups within a profession, which may mean that the end result is homogenous, bland and not very alternative. Any attempt to devise profession-wide competencies must try to ensure that as many therapeutic groups are consulted as possible.

The point of defining competencies is that they represent agreement within the therapy as to what constitute the core elements of being able to practise that therapy in a safe and effective manner. Different training schools will continue to provide their own, even idiosyncratic, approach to training which will continue to promote diversity within each profession. The establishment of core competencies is nonetheless important to be able to consolidate and promote cohesion and to set out the minimum requirements for training and practice. However difficult it may be to arrive at competencies which can be agreed across an entire profession, both consumers and regulators could legitimately express concern if practitioners within a given therapy cannot agree on what competencies are necessary for the safe and effective practice of that therapy.

Can holistic therapies be broken down into competencies?

Some therapists argue that an approach which is holistic and intuitive cannot be broken down into a set of definable competencies, as these will inevitably fail to capture the essence of the therapeutic encounter and will make their encounters with patients mechanical. The technical aspects of training cannot necessarily be pinned down in a set of step-by-step actions. This would be unrealistic and an insult to the professional autonomy of the practitioner applying technical knowledge. For this reason, many licensing boards do not specify the technical content of the course, but require certain numbers of theoretical and practical training hours instead. What *can* be described are the non-technical aspects of work. The following competencies included in the UK's *National Occupational Standards for Hypnotherapy*[2] provide examples of the sorts of core competencies which might need to be addressed.

* Promoting patient's equality diversity and rights.
* Exploring, evaluating and reviewing with patients the goals of therapy.
* Structuring, implementing and reviewing treatment.

- Monitoring and adapting content, approach and technique as necessary.
- Facilitating the patient's understanding and ability to effect change within themselves.
- Evaluating, prioritising and reviewing overall workload.
- Promoting effective communication and relationships.
- Promoting, monitoring and maintaining health, safety and security in the workplace.
- Developing knowledge and practice.
- Contributing to the development of knowledge and practice of others.
- Enabling individuals to address issues which affect their health and social well-being.
- Supporting individuals when they are distressed.

Do formalised competencies stultify individual style?

The concern is that if professional bodies define competencies too rigidly, this may inadvertently stultify members' practice – although therapies which have produced formal competencies would disagree with this point. The argument against introducing rigid competencies is that this is thought to inhibit the individual practitioner's style and creativity. What is at stake is the personal freedom of each individual practitioner to work as he or she sees fit, and whether this professional autonomy can or should be restricted for the sake of patient safety and the good of the profession as a whole. This is felt to be a particular issue for alternative therapists, who pride themselves on the individual perspective they bring to their work. Many CAM therapists eschew the homogenised processing of patients which they think characterises allopathic, symptom-orientated medicine and reject top-down hierarchies and the work-based competencies they promote.

How far can alternative practitioners reject being part of a collective? Depending on licensing requirements, a practitioner may choose to work entirely independently, rejecting formal training and refusing to belong to a professional association. How much credibility such a person could have would be debatable, as is their right to term themselves as a 'health practitioner'. Farsides argues that the maintenance of professional standards requires practitioners to accept the guidance and control of their regulators.[3] She suggests that individual professional autonomy must be compatible with concepts of obedience and co-operation. But as Farsides's analysis reveals, another way of looking at professional autonomy is to consider its link with the issue of responsibility. Being ultimately and solely responsible for decisions one makes is another way of interpreting autonomy. Thus, she argues:

> A claim for independence or control, which is so often at the heart of ideas of self-rule, must also entail the acceptance of responsibility if it is to carry moral weight.[4]

Issues of accountability and professional responsibility are implicit in this understanding of professional autonomy. In terms of safeguarding the public, an obvious question is how willing practitioners would be to exercise accountability in thinking about the above issues in the absence of defined competencies and professional structures? Until training standards are consistently high, nationally defined competencies might be a means of ensuring practitioners work to an acceptable standard.

Making realistic claims

A competent CAM practitioner must be realistic about the claims that are made to patients. Much of the medical profession's hostility towards CAM therapists arises because of the inflated claims made. Pantanowitz insists:

> False claims cause all the trouble. False claims will not prevent sickness and death. They will delay patients in getting to the doctor, who may indeed be able to treat the sickness and prevent untimely death. Alternative practitioners must not be allowed to make false claims and sell false hope.[5]

Although this quote masks a number of hidden assumptions (what counts as evidence; should CAM be avoided where there is a conventional alternative; whether the patients subjective experience of hope is 'false hope', etc.), the sentiment is widely shared. Clearly CAM treatment can bring about significant health benefits for some patients. In the absence of research, practitioners should avoid making over-optimistic claims about what a therapy can deliver. Most professional codes explicitly discourage their members from creating false expectations or guaranteeing a cure.

Recognising limits of competence

Therapists need to recognise when a clinical situation is beyond the realms of their competence. The individual and isolated context in which many practitioners work makes this a particularly acute issue. Most therapists work on their own and once they have qualified they may have little contact with their training organisation, with other therapists working in the same discipline, or with their professional registering body. It is useful to contrast this model with the hierarchical way in which most doctors work. As Sharma describes:

They work in the context of medical bureaucracies and their responsibilities to their employers and to other doctors cannot be ignored.[6]

Working within this sort of organisational context facilitates wide-ranging systems of delegation and referral, which allows patients to access the widest possible range of professional expertise. Although a small proportion of CAM practitioners work within a group practice setting, Sharma's research found that, unlike most doctors, the majority of CAM practitioners work as self-employed, freelance professionals whose income is proportionate to the number of patients they see. She notes:

A characteristic of some of the therapists was a positive distaste for working within a large organisation, a desire to have control over one's working conditions even at the expense of security. This was particularly true of some therapists who had formerly worked in the NHS (usually as nurses) and were appreciative of the greater therapeutic autonomy they felt they enjoyed as independent practitioners.

Ethically, this aspect of CAM raises potential concerns over safety and accountability. Sharma continues:

Complementary therapists, therefore, tend to work in settings characterised by a non-hierarchical ethos and minimum of direct control from either superiors or equals. Thus they appear to have the clinical autonomy and freedom from managerial interference which doctors hold as an ideal, but without the control exercised by professional colleagues which doctors also hold to be the main safeguard against poor standards of practice. Indeed this apparent conjunction of liberty and non-accountability may explain the particularly hostile attitude which some orthodox doctors entertain towards complementary practitioners.[7]

This is not to suggest that complementary practitioners deliberately expose their patients to harm. Problems may arise where practitioners do not even realise (or acknowledge) that they are out of their depth. Where there are no colleagues with whom a problematic case can be discussed, a practitioner is more likely to proceed with treatment, albeit on a cautious basis. This lack of any clear managerial structure highlights why effective supervision is necessary to protect patients.

Making effective referrals

These problems are compounded by the absence of any clear referral structures. This manifests in three areas:

1   referrals from one therapist to another therapist working within the same therapy, for example, from one osteopath to another osteopath;
2   referrals from one therapist to a therapist working in another therapeutic discipline, for example, from an osteopath to an acupuncturist;
3   referrals from CAM practitioners to a GP or other conventional physician.

Referrals of the first kind may be hampered by therapists' needing to make a living and their unwillingness to lose a client. A homoeopath trying to build up a client base is unlikely to send the patient to another homoeopath who might be better able to relieve the patient's problems. Additionally, the absence of a career progression within complementary medicine means that inexperienced therapists do not have the option of sending a patient to a consultant or specialist within their own therapy. They would only be able to recommend a more experienced practitioner whom they happened to know of personally or through word of mouth. Financial factors may also operate in the second kind of referral, although therapists are equally likely to be constrained by a genuine lack of knowledge about other therapies. Even if a chiropractor had a general understanding about homoeopathy and acupuncture, there is little comparative research between these complete systems, so there is little way of saying with any certainty which approach would best benefit the patient.

Referrals of the third kind are restrained by cultural barriers and regulatory barriers, which will only be broken down by greater openness and integration. Some doctors are dismissive of alternative medicine, and are hostile to patients who consult complementary practitioners. A survey conducted in 1992 by Sharma found that only a minority (30 per cent) of interviewees had told their GP that they were using non-orthodox medicine. Leaving aside issues of confidentiality, unless constructive dialogue can be established, therapists are unlikely to interface directly with a patient's GP or conventional doctor. This can be potentially disastrous if the patient has an existing pathology which requires urgent conventional treatment.

To what extent, if any, should CAM practitioners ensure that the patient seeks a medical opinion before undertaking therapy? Suggesting that all patients need to see a doctor before consulting a therapist would clearly be excessive and unworkable. This would also dramatically limit the scope of a CAM practitioner to diagnose and treat the patient within an alternative paradigm. However, failing to refer a patient to a physician in circumstances in which a reasonable practitioner would refer could find the CAM practitioner subject to legal or disciplinary procedures. A middle ground, in which practitioners refer their patients to a physician *where appropriate*, requires sufficient knowledge of anatomy, physiology and conventional diagnostics to be included in the CAM curriculum. Deciding how much medical information is necessary is extremely difficult and will vary from therapy to therapy. Moreover, there may be situations where CAM therapists will treat acute medical conditions within their own diagnostic framework, situations in which doctors would feel that urgent conventional treatment ought to be given, as the following case study demonstrates:

> *An experienced homoeopath is widely known in his local area for being radically opposed to conventional medicine. On two occasions, his professional body has received complaints against him from a local GP who claims that he has countermanded his own instructions to patients by telling them to throw away their antibiotics. Accordingly, when a long-standing patient of the homoeopath presents with a high temperature and severe swelling in his arm, the homoeopath diagnoses cellulitis and, with the patient's consent, proceeds to treat the condition homoeopathically. Because of the severity of this condition, the homoeopath makes two house calls to the patient in a three-day period and telephones four times a day for a week to monitor his condition. The patient makes a full recovery. Some months later, he attends his GP's surgery for a pre-employment medical. When the patient discloses that he had cellulitis successfully treated by the homoeopath, the GP is furious. He telephones the homoeopath's professional body insisting that it is a wonder that his patient didn't die and asserting that at the very least, the homoeopath should have had the courtesy to inform the patient's GP of his condition. He demands that the homoeopath be struck off for failure to refer.*

Certainly, this case study demonstrates the difficulties when there is a discrepancy between how a CAM practitioner would choose to diagnose and manage a treatment episode and how a conventional doctor might have acted in similar circumstances. This case study also draws attention to the difficulties caused by poor communication. There is a difference, however, between appropriately trained CAM therapists who realise the severity of a patient's condition and who arrive at a clinical judgement that the condition can be treated within their own diagnostic framework, and inadequately trained practitioners who simply fail to appreciate the severity of a patient's condition. Provided a full explanation had been given and consent has been sought, CAM practitioners would not be liable for treating an acute illness for which treatment exists within their diagnostic framework, even if there was not a good therapeutic outcome – although, arguably, there may be a duty to refer to a conventional practitioner if the CAM therapy is not working and the patient's condition is becoming critical. The UK government has stated:

Diagnostic procedures must be reliable and reproducible and more attention must be paid to whether CAM diagnostic procedures, as well as CAM therapies, have been scientifically validated.[8]

However, the countervailing ethical consideration is that the therapist must respect the patient's autonomy and a patient cannot be forced to seek orthodox medial treatment. Many therapists treat patients who have explicitly rejected orthodox treatment. This does not absolve the practitioner, ethically or legally, from knowing when the patient is suffering from a serious pathology and from *advising* the patient to seek medical attention where appropriate. Such discussions should always be recorded in the patient's notes. Occasionally, a practitioner may feel that it would be inappropriate to continue to treat a patient who refuses to consult a conventional practitioner. Nonetheless, therapists should respect the duty of confidentiality they owe their patients and should not consult the patient's physician without their consent unless there is an exceptional reason to do so.

Collaboration with other health professionals

No one therapist, conventional or alternative, has the skills and experience to treat every patient who seeks help. The need to work alongside other practitioners, or to refer patients to a more appropriate practitioner, is a central requirement of justice as well as beneficent practice. As the benefits of CAM become increasingly recognised, the flow of patients between conventional and complementary practitioners will become more commonplace. Featherstone and Forsyth state:

> To refer patients to another health care professional – if that practitioner will be better suited to help them to improve their health – is the only ethical thing to do. Structures of professional relationships and communication need to be established which will allow access and movement across the boundaries of orthodox and complementary medicine. This has to become the norm within modern health care systems if patients are to be provided with the support they clearly want.[9]

Greater collaboration between CAM practitioners and other health professionals would benefit patients, who would be treated by the therapist most able to offer benefit to them. For CAM practitioners, greater collaboration may provide access to state funding, opportunities to conduct effective research, and the wider availability of their therapies. Many doctors appreciate that greater collaboration with CAM practitioners may improve patient care by providing options to groups of patients for whom conventional medicine has little to offer, for example, patients suffering from stress-related disorders, musculo-skeletal problems and persistent pain; by allowing doctors to develop an increased awareness of interactions between conventional and alternative treatments; and by freeing doctors up to spend more time with patients who require or prefer a conventional approach to care.

For greater collaboration to exist, CAM practitioners must have familiarisation with conventional diagnostics and treatments, and conventional practitioners must have far greater awareness of available CAM treatments. The UK government has recently supported greater familiarisation for conventional health professionals at both under-graduate and post-graduate levels. It draws a crucial distinction between courses aimed at providing conventional practitioners with some familiarisation in CAM for the purpose of advising patients, and courses intended to equip practitioners to offer CAM treatments themselves. In the latter case, the government supports the training of conventional health care practitioners to standards agreed with an appropriate (single) CAM regulatory body.[10]

'Whole' systems

Whole systems of health and healing, such as acupuncture, herbalism, homoeopathy and Ayurveda, are perceived to be more of a threat by orthodox medical practitioners than therapeutic or diagnostic techniques, such as aromatherapy or iridology. This is because whole disciplines provide a unified theory which can account for all illness, thus increasing the likelihood of a patient failing to seek orthodox medical treatment where this is indicated. Fortunately, the risk is minimised because practitioners of 'whole therapies' tend to have a lengthier training and to be more intensely regulated than practitioners of other CAM therapies used in a more adjuvant fashion. Nonetheless, therapists who have such a broad array of therapeutic options within their modality may feel that there is always something they could do to benefit a given patient. From an ethical point of view, the concern is not so much that this is a false claim, rather that the overly zealous practitioner is less likely to refer the patient to another therapist or doctor who could benefit the patient more.

Cross-specialisation

The competence of CAM practitioners may be called into question when a practitioner who is trained in one therapy incorporates techniques from another therapy. It is very common for therapists to use a variety of therapeutic modalities when treating clients. Vincent and Furnham note:

> Complementary practitioners, although usually having one major specialty, may use, comment on and recommend a very wide range of different treatment methods in routine clinical practice. The most

widely used supplementary regimes are diet, exercise, vitamins, herbal remedies, massage and relaxation. These are core treatments drawn on by many practitioners. [11]

Perhaps it is in the nature of treating patients holistically that therapists are comfortable with the idea of incorporating new therapeutic tools into their work. CAM therapists, unlike doctors, do not categorise illness within a reductionist framework and thus do not limit their work to specialisations and sub-specialisations. The high level of professional autonomy that therapists enjoy means that they are free to incorporate new and different therapeutic skills without having to seek permission.

Use of more than one therapeutic approach is ethically acceptable *provided* practitioners are adequately trained in each of the disciplines they are using. As a matter of public safety, it would not, for example, be acceptable for an osteopath to attend a couple of weekend courses in acupuncture and then start incorporating acupuncture into his or her practice. Ideally, before offering any therapy, all practitioners (be they conventional or alternative) should have a relevant qualification in that area based on theoretical knowledge and practical experience. If this is not the case, at the very least, practitioners must make it clear to the patient that this is not their main area of expertise and should be able to make a referral to a practitioner who is fully trained in that field.

Assessing the competence of traditionally trained CAM practitioners

As CAM has become more professionalised over the last years, training has been incorporated into higher education systems, and many CAM practitioners study at diploma or degree level. There is a shift away from private training schools towards externally accredited college/university-based training. Many courses provide an academic training alongside a practical training and students may gain hands-on experience through teaching clinics attached to these institutions. These developments are seen as part of the move towards professionalisation and as a necessary precondition to integration with conventional medicine.

Yet, the higher education approach to training is not necessarily the best, or indeed, only effective way of training competent CAM practitioners. The cultural context of the therapy may have a significant impact on how new therapists are initiated or inducted into practice. Cassidy compares the training systems favoured by professionalised systems with the way in which practitioners learn their craft in community-based systems:

> Found in both urban and rural settings, training is often by apprenticeship. People enter training sometimes by inheritance, but most

often by receiving a call from the unseen world indicating that he or she has the special capacity necessary to become a healer. Training ends when the teacher considers the student to be ready to practice. Rather than written examinations, students are tested by practising under guidance: essentially, the community itself determines if a student is 'good enough'.[12]

Apprenticeship models are unlikely to find favour in western nations committed to tertiary education. But, as the above quote indicates, a formal education may not be sufficient to guarantee that a graduate is competent to treat patients. Whilst much of a practitioner's technical knowledge may be gained at a pre-registration level, the practical skills and wisdom required of a competent practitioner may take months or years of practical experience to accumulate. Training needs to be seen as the beginning of the process, and not the end point. Education should be seen not as a one-off, but a life-long learning process. There are various mechanisms by which this can be achieved. These can include provisional periods of practice before qualifying as a fully registered practitioner, continuous professional development (CPD), research and revalidation.

Notes

1 Palmer Barnes, P. (1998) *Complaints and Grievances in Psychotherapy. A Handbook of Ethical Practice.* Routledge: London and New York.
2 Care Sector Consortium (1999) *National Occupational Standards for Hypnotherapy.* Other sets of standards have been devised for aromatherapy, reflexology and homoeopathy, but none have not been widely taken up at the time of writing.
3 Farsides, C. (1994) 'Autonomy, Responsibility and Midwifery'. In Budd, S. and Sharma, U. (eds) *The Healing Bond.* Routledge: London and New York.
4 Ibid., 51.
5 Pantanowitz, D. (1994) *Alternative Medicine. A Doctor's Perspective.* Southern Book Publishers.
6 Sharma, U. (1994) 'The Equation of Responsibility. Complementary Practitioners and Their Patients'. In Budd, S. and Sharma, U., op. cit.
7 Ibid.
8 *Government's Response to the House of Lords Select Committee on Science and Technology's Report on Complementary and Alternative Medicine* (2001). The Stationery Office: London.
9 Featherstone, C. and Forsyth, L. (1997) *Medical Marriage: The New Partnership Between Orthodox and Complementary Medicine.* Findhorn Press: Findhorn, Scotland.
10 *Government's Response to the House of Lords Select Committee,* op. cit.
11 Vincent, C. and Furnham, A. (1997) *Complementary Medicine. A Research Perspective.* John Wiley & Sons: Chichester, Chapter 1.
12 Cassidy, C.M. (1996) 'Cultural Context of Complementary and Alternative Medicine Systems'. In Micozzi, M. (ed.) *Fundamentals of Complementary and Alternative Medicine.* Churchill Livingstone: Edinburgh.

8

RESEARCH

Key ethical issues:
* Political dimensions of CAM research
* Implications for CAM of evidence-based medicine
* Exploring the barriers to CAM research
* Conducting research and obtaining ethical review
* Practical ways to make clinical practice more effective

Research: the political agenda

The research debate within CAM is probably the most controversial and politically important issue affecting therapists. The shortage of credible scientific evidence to support the use of CAM has been used as a political stick to justify CAM's continued exclusion from state-funded health systems. There is, however, an increasing amount of evidence to support the use of CAM in a variety of clinical situations. There is also a large body of evidence from non-western countries supporting the use of traditional therapies, but this is largely disregarded by western research communities. The purpose of this book is not to evaluate the quality of the evidence underpinning CAM practice, but to consider the ethical issues raised by CAM research. This necessarily involves discussion of both the political dimensions of CAM research as well as the ethics of conducting effective research.

The argument against integrating CAM at the present time is its lack of evidence base and a perceived unwillingness amongst some practitioners to submit CAM techniques to scientific scrutiny. Doctors argue that if conventional medicine has to demonstrate that its techniques are effective, it is fair to demand that complementary and alternative therapies should be tested with similar rigour. Herein lies the main area of contention. Many of those who argue that CAM must be validated before it is provided as part of a state-funded system would like to see the same scientific methods used to demonstrate efficacy of conventional medicine being applied to CAM techniques. An obvious example is proposing that product-based therapies (for example, herbal and homoeopathy remedies) should be tested by means of the randomised control trials (RCTs) used to test allopathic medicines. Many practitioners now concede that CAM therapies should be tested, but insist that this requires methodology which is appropriate to CAM practice.

A concern felt by therapists is that the entire framework underpinning medical research is based on the predominating biomedical paradigm, using concepts of health and disease, cause and effect, and extrapolations from the general population to the individual, which do not capture the holistic experience. Cohen analyses the medical reaction to this sentiment as an attack on scientism. He observes:

> Holistic modalities by and large do not purport to diagnose and treat pathology as it is defined within the biomedical paradigm, and thus do not rely wholly for validation on the double-blind, randomized studies that are published in peer-reviewed journals following the scientific principles accepted within dominant medical circles. On the other hand, many holistic modalities do involve repeated observations, measurement and comparison of results over multiple generations searching for unifying principles.[1]

What Cohen is suggesting is that CAM practitioners are already concerned with outcomes and use empirical methods, albeit in a non-systematic way. Even within therapies where there is not much recognised scientific literature, it would be an absurd misrepresentation to suggest that therapists do not base their treatment on an accumulation of knowledge gained through the mechanisms Cohen describes. As self-employed practitioners, CAM therapists have to be concerned with patient outcomes and patient satisfaction, without necessarily being particularly 'research-minded'. One solution to bridge this divide is to reconsider what is meant by the term 'scientific' research. Cohen continues:

> Many providers advocate an epistemology of science which includes phenomenological and experiential data and thus addresses 'the totality of the human experience'.[2]

This echoes Eskinazi's definition of CAM discussed previously, which points out that CAM challenges the definition and parameters of science itself. Rather than dismissing CAM research as insufficiently scientific, the scientific community may be forced to reconsider the whole question of what ought to count as proof. This shift is already reflected in qualitative research studies now being carried out, and the growing attention given to patient-centred outcomes.[3] This is an important point for therapists to realise, since many therapists may have an unrealistic picture about what constitutes clinical research. This may put them off conducting simple research within their own practice, even though this could significantly improve their professional development as well as their external profile.

The reluctance to conduct research may not, however, be due to obstinacy or lack or research skills on the part of CAM therapists, but may reveal a much more fundamental difference between how CAM therapists and conventional doctors view the world. As Fulder observes:

> There is [within alternative medicine] a lack of urgency to construct explanatory models – an empiricism incorporating a greater sense of the unknown and respect that goes with it.[4]

The question of what counts as *good enough* evidence is highly political and cannot be divorced from the extent to which scientific knowledge is exalted in the western world above all other forms of knowledge. As Cassidy points out:

> Euroamerican society in particular has developed science to be the believable knowledge method, the knowledge orthodoxy of the late nineteenth and twentieth centuries. The determination with which Westerners cling to their cultural preference concerning the power of science approaches a religious fervour.[5]

The argument that CAM therapies should conduct *scientific* research may be masking a value-laden cultural preference for the scientific method and its ability to reveal 'the truth'. In comparison, any other means of demonstrating the effectiveness of alternative systems will be taken to have less validity. Cassidy continues:

> Given that the other major systems are not experimental – they depend on well-developed clinical observation skills and experience guided by their explanatory models – it becomes clear why a system that perceives itself as scientific can consider non-scientific systems as inferior in our cultural milieu.[6]

Because of the shortage of research expertise amongst CAM practitioners, much of the research which has been conducted and published has been criticised for being of poor quality, and even research which has shown CAM to have positive effects has been accused of lacking scientific rigour. Although more therapists are interested in doing research than in the past, some therapists are still reluctant to invest precious time and money in empirical research *merely* to pander to that sector of the medical profession who will not take them seriously unless such evidence exists.

The reluctance to conduct research may be particularly strong in therapies which have a long history of safe usage and with which patients appear to be satisfied. This argument is frequently advanced in relation to herbal medicine and acupuncture. This position is ethically unsustainable. The duty to benefit and not harm patients requires all therapies to be *as safe as possible*. Traditional usage may provide *prima facie* evidence as to the safety of a therapy, but may not answer some of the questions that users of CAM therapies need to know in order to make informed choices. Research comparing the use of different therapeutic interventions in patients suffering from a particular condition would be particularly beneficial to patients uncertain which therapy is the most appropriate for them at that point. Patients should be able to make their choice on the basis of good information, and in many therapies that knowledge does not yet exist. The fact that patients have not been deterred by a lack of evidence can no longer be considered a good reason not to attempt to answer these questions.

For this knowledge to become available, CAM practitioners must be personally prepared to become involved in research. This does not mean that all practitioners should give up their clinical practice and devote themselves to undertaking large-scale clinical trials. But, all practitioners should be carrying out some form of empirical validation of their work. Many practitioners will be doing this already. All practitioners already draw on and build on their previous experience to validate their own therapeutic approach and refine their own techniques. But as Canter and Nanke point out:

> Though such personal conviction may be valuable to the individual clinician and their patients, it is of little help in contributing to collective, dependable knowledge about the process of effects of different types of therapy. This requires systematic empirical investigation, producing objective results which can be evaluated by others within the discipline and the wider scientific community.[7]

The rise of evidence-based medicine

Prompted by concerns over the quality and consistency of medical treatment, the fear of being sued and the need to demonstrate value for money, state-funded health providers have become committed to the concept of evidence-based medicine. In the past, much conventional medicine drew on expert intuition and unvalidated custom and practice, leading to an unacceptable variation in treatment rates and the extent to which practitioners integrated patient's values into their choice of treatment.

The purpose of evidence-based medicine is to ensure that decisions about the care of individual patients is based on 'conscientious, explicit and judicious use of current best evidence'.[8] As Kerridge *et al.* note:

> Evidence based medicine is based on a strong ethical and clinical ideal – that it allows the best evaluated methods of health care to be

identified and enables patients and doctors to make better informed decisions.[9]

Although there may be difficulties in its implementation, it is vital to appreciate the beneficence-based ideal which underpins evidence-based practice. Davidoff *et al.* identify five issues central to evidence-based practice:

- clinical decisions should be based on the best available scientific evidence;
- the clinical problem – rather than the habit of protocols – should determine the type of evidence to be sought;
- identifying the best evidence means using epidemiological and biostatistical ways of thinking;
- conclusions derived from identifying and critically appraising evidence are useful only if put into action in managing patients or making health care decisions;
- performance should be constantly evaluated.[10]

Clinicians' main objection to evidence-based medicine is that it suppresses clinical freedom. But Sackett *et al.* stress:

> The practice of evidence-based medicine means integrating individual clinical expertise with the best available external clinical evidence from systematic research.... Good doctors use both individual clinical expertise and the best available evidence, and neither alone is enough.[11]

As well as fearing the loss of their individual professional autonomy, some practitioners believe that evidence-based medicine is detrimental to individualised, patient-centred care and will result in formulaic treatment. Yet the decision whether the evidence applies to the particular patient, and if so, how this should translate into a clinical decision, remains an important function of the individual practitioner's expertise. This is important, since treatments which appear to be beneficial in a research setting may be of negligible benefit in a real-life situation, and, in the real world, practitioners have to work intuitively and subjectively. Greenhalgh argues that an intuitive and subjective approach is not inconsistent with evidence-based practice:

> Far from obviating the need for subjectivity in the clinical encounter, genuine evidence based practice actually presupposes an interpretive paradigm in which the patient experiences illness in a unique and contextual way. Furthermore, it is only within an interpretive paradigm that a clinician can meaningfully draw on all

aspects of evidence – his or her own care based experience, the patient's individual and cultural preferences, and the results of rigorous clinical research trials and observational studies – to reach an integrated clinical judgment.[12]

Within evidence-based CAM, the role of the practitioner in applying the evidence to the particular case will be enhanced, not hindered, by the extent to which CAM practitioners attempt to understand their patient's interpretation of their illness and to respect their patient's values.

Evidence-based practice is perceived to operate against CAM because many therapies lack evidence in the form of randomised controlled trials (RCTs) or meta-analyses (which combine the results of all available RCTs). The biomedical hierarchy of evidence has operated to exclude many studies of CAM in the past, and particularly personal anecdotes, on the basis that they are of an insufficient standard to be regarded as scientifically worthwhile. Evidence-based medicine operates at a threshold below which evidence is considered so poor as not to be worth considering in most situations.[13]

As evidence-based practice draws on the best available evidence, CAM practitioners should not be deterred from working towards evidence-based practice in the absence of RCTs, but should draw on such research data as are currently available. At the same time, the strength of evidence-based clinical decisions will depend on the quality and relevance of the evidence and on its interpretation. As such, the onus is on CAM researchers to confront the difficulties posed by evidence-based medicine by working towards developing research methodologies which can yield generalisable data, but at the same time, contribute to decision-making involving individual patients. The inclusion of qualitative measures will assist this process.

The political influence of evidence-based medicine cannot be overlooked. Governments and health funders are attracted to the idea of allocating health resources on the basis of evidence. Resources will be directed towards those areas of health care which are demonstrable by evidence and away from interventions which have not been proven to be efficacious. This means that evidence-based health care has an inherent bias against therapeutic interventions in which outcomes cannot be adequately measured or easily defined, such as psychotherapy or healing. Moreover, doctors and pharmaceutical companies often determine the research agenda, so that evidence is most likely to support drug-based interventions rather than alternative or multi-faceted approaches, for which there may be less evidence available.

Medicine is now heavily influenced by evidence-based culture. For reasons discussed, integration of CAM and conventional medicine is likely to take the form of CAM being incorporated into the dominant medical framework. This means that CAM will be integrated into an evidence-based medical culture, which will demand that individual treatment decisions be taken in the light of the best available evidence. As Lewith *et al.* predict:

> If we are to develop an integrated approach that will allow us to combine the best of conventional medicine and complementary and alternative medicine in order to provide an informed choice for our patients, then it must be research led and evidence based.[14]

Whilst a commitment to research is a collective responsibility of all CAM practitioners, and will be crucial if CAM is to attract government funding, not all practitioners will be suited to conducting *formal* clinical research, and other practitioners may find it more productive to direct their energies towards monitoring their own clinical practice and carrying out audits or small scale studies on their own or in collaboration with a small group of colleagues. The Research Council for Complementary Medicine's website (information@rccm.organisation.uk) provides invaluable assistance to therapists trying to decide what level of research is suitable for them. The remainder of this section will first look at formal research into CAM and the problems associated with it, and then consider less formal approaches which all practitioners can incorporate into their practice.

Conducting formal CAM research

CAM research needs to answer five salient questions, identified by Vincent and Furnham (these will be of varying importance depending on the developmental stage of a therapy and what research has already been carried out). The questions they identify are:

- Does the therapy have a beneficial effect on any individual disease or disorder?
- Does the treatment have any advantage over existing treatments in terms of efficacy, safety, patient preference, cost and availability?
- Is this effect primarily, or even partly, due to the specific and intended action of the treatment as opposed to placebo?
- What mechanism might underlie the therapy's actions?
- What are the process issues around the reliability and validity of diagnosis, the value of individual techniques, the role of the practitioner and the attitude of the patient. [15]

These larger research questions can only really be answered by means of well-designed, formal clinical research trials. These need to be undertaken by practitioners who already have experience of trial design, conduct, analysis and interpretation of data. Clinical researchers will also need experience in submitting applications for funding and seeking ethical approval for their study (discussed below).

Practical and methodological difficulties in carrying out CAM research

Although a stronger CAM research culture is beginning to emerge, there are still significant practical and methodological problems which hamper CAM research. These include the following:

- Lack of research skills, previously not prioritised in CAM therapists' training, together with lack of career development opportunities/funded posts for CAM practitioners who wish to specialise in research.
- Isolation of working in sole practice, reducing the likelihood of collaborative research, compounded by lack of external or institutional pressure to conduct research.
- Therapists perceiving treating patients and earning a living as higher priorities than committing time to (probably unfunded) research.
- Difficulties in finding sufficient numbers of (fee-paying) CAM patients who are prepared to be research subjects and are prepared to be randomised.
- Difficulties in designing appropriate research methodologies to measure highly individualised treatments. Problems may be compounded by the absence of standardisation of product-based remedies. Research may be even harder in therapies where the underlying mechanism is not yet understood.
- Difficulties in getting research funding and apparent bias against CAM researchers.[16]
- Publication bias against CAM research on the part of mainstream medical journals.[17]
- Lack of knowledge on the part of ethical review boards as to how to deal with protocols involving different conceptual frameworks.
- Problem that the research carried out and published tends to be by medical practitioners within a biomedicalised research framework.
- Lack of appropriate environments and management skills for running CAM trials (accordingly, research being limited to a few centres of excellence).

These problems have been well documented and have undoubtedly hindered research in the past.[18] However, there has also been an unfortunate tendency to conflate all these difficulties. As a result, many practitioners are apathetic towards conducting research. This is regrettable, since the more good quality research is conducted, the more willing funders will be to support further research and the stronger the impetus will be for journals to publish. There may, however, be little that individual practitioners can do to overcome some of these impediments to conducting wide-scale research. Fostering a strong research culture imposes collective responsibilities on professional bodies and training establishments.

Devising appropriate research methodologies

Much of the discussion about CAM research focusses on the vexed question of trial design and of finding reproducible ways of demonstrating that CAM interventions are effective, centring on the unsuitability of RCTs to determine whether CAM works. The RCT represents the 'gold standard' of clinical research. The main objection to applying RCTs to CAM is that they are not appropriate for measuring therapies which are individualistic in nature, which may involve multiple interventions, and which do not have an immediate causal effect on symptoms.

Although many practitioners do not appreciate this, RCTs do not require that all research subjects receive standardised treatment. Pragmatic RCTs may be a useful trial design, since these combine rigorous methodology with all of the variables of therapists' actual, clinical practice. As Vincent and Furnham point out, whilst the difficulties of applying conventional method-ologies to CAM are real, this has not hindered research in other areas where practitioners have to exercise considerable subjective judgement, for example, psychotherapy or even surgery.[19] If it is felt that RCTs do not capture the holistic experience, the onus is on CAM researchers to develop methodologies which are better able to encapsulate the individual variations within therapeutic practice.

Controlled trials present problems to CAM therapists, since they obscure the differences between patients, particularly in relation to an individual's treatment response. Whilst this is an issue which lies in part with the trial design, it also highlights a fundamental problem with research. Research can never replicate the complexities of a clinical setting. Research findings will inevitably be in generalised terms. Research trials do tend to look at groups of patients rather than at individuals, because the research question inevitably poses a broad question, namely: 'Is this treatment *generally* bene-ficial for this condition.'[20] Research findings can never provide the definitive answer as to how an individual patient should be treated or how an indi-vidual patient will respond to treatment. That decision will always rest with the individual practitioner, who remains accountable for treatment decisions.

Many CAM practitioners feel that patient satisfaction ought to be enough to confer credibility on a practice, whereas the scientific community place more reliance on objective, rather than subjective, outcome measures. Practitioners might be heartened to appreciate the extent to which the patient's subjective experience is of increasing importance in all areas of health care research. Even pharmaceutical drug trials now attempt to elicit the patient's response, including qualitative measures alongside quantitative dimensions of a research protocol. This information is now not only regarded as desirable, but also as scientifically respectable. [21]

Even within CAM though, patient-centred outcomes can be enhanced by more objective measures. There are many clinical situations within CAM where objective outcome measures can be applied. Objective measurements can be made, for example, in trials of hypertension, eczema or joint mobility which do not depend on the patient's interpretation of their symptoms but can be objectively measured by researchers, thus adding to the findings' reliability and reproducibility.

Another focus of concern involves the therapist's subjective interpretation of patient measures. The argument is that subjectivity renders measures such as the acupuncturists' pulse taking or the iridologist's observation of the iris too variable to be meaningful. Yet the subjectivity inherent in these measures does not mean that they are inherently unacceptable, merely that their reliability and validity needs to be established, as with any other outcome measurement. Investigating the value of the indicator is separate from evaluating the treatment itself, so that acupuncture may be valuable even if the pulse approach is unreliable. This is critical, because significant practitioner bias will prevent a patient from receiving the best treatment. Johannessen illustrates this point in her research of practitioners in Denmark:

> In the clinics I visited, it was obvious that each practitioner worked along personal patterns of diagnosis and prescription. One kinesiologist, for example, diagnosed malfunctioning pancreas in 16 of the 26 patients whose treatment I observed, while this particular problem was not diagnosed in any of the 19 patients of another kinesiologist. [22]

Whilst the extent of therapist/patient interaction is such that sham treatments may not be practical (particularly in massage, manipulative or talking therapies) and the placebo effect may be significant, systematic review of patient consultations ought nonetheless to reveal unacceptable levels of practitioner preferences.

Submitting research proposals to a research ethics committee

Most countries require any research involving human subjects to undergo ethical review. In the UK, all research which takes place on NHS premises, or involves NHS patients, has to be submitted to a research ethics committee (REC). In the US, there are similar requirements for research on human subjects to be approved by an Institutional Review Board (IRB). The function of ethics committees is to ensure that the proposed research is both scientifically sound (since bad design is bad ethics) and, more significantly, that the rights of the research subjects are not compromised in order to obtain the results sought. In the UK, ethical review is only mandatory for research involving NHS patients. Because most CAM encounters operate in the private sector, there is no obligation for CAM research to be scrutinised by a research ethics committee. This should not deter CAM researchers from seeking ethical review in any event. The benefits of submitting research to an independent ethics committee include:

- ensuring that the research is not only ethical, but is seen to be so by the public;
- reassurance that the researcher is not the sole arbiter in deciding whether the research is ethical;
- most peer-reviewed journals will not accept research articles for publication unless the researchers have obtained ethical approval for the study;
- funding bodies are reluctant to fund research that has not been approved by an independent research ethics committee;
- the need to present the research for ethical review will focus the mind of researchers on both methodology (will the design of the research be capable of yielding answers to the questions posed?) and ethical issues (are the rights of research subjects being adequately protected?);
- an increase in CAM applications to ethics committees will heighten awareness of CAM's prevalence and force ethics committees to consider what amounts to 'good' science and whether ethics committees are appropriately constituted to be able to judge the merits of CAM protocols.

Most review boards have only limited experience of processing CAM applications, although most ethics committees are increasingly presented with studies which are either based wholly on qualitative research, or which combine qualitative and quantitative methodology. As well as trial design, other key aspects of ethical review are the consent of the research subject, the confidentiality of the data and the acceptability of the risk/benefit ratio involved in participation. These will be explored in turn.

Consent to participate in research

Provided the ethics committee is satisfied that the trial design is capable of yielding the information sought, the next ethical concern is that research subjects should be given fully informed consent to take part in the research. As with any treatment, the rationale for this requirement is that people should not be exposed to any degree of risk, however slight, unless they have so consented. This is especially relevant in relation to non-therapeutic research, where the subject is not even anticipated to benefit directly from the trial. Usually, the consent will be in writing and needs to be recorded in the patient's medical records. Most research projects fail to satisfy the ethical review process because the consent or patient information provisions are felt to be inadequate. Patient information needs to include the following:

- the fact that subjects are participating in a trial;
- what the trial is attempting to prove;
- what the risks will be to the trial subject and what the treatment alternatives are;
- an assurance that subjects are free to withdraw from the study at any point;
- a guarantee that their treatment will not be compromised in any way if they withdraw from the trial, or choose not to participate;
- information as to compensation should they be harmed as a result of inclusion in the study;
- a name of someone whom research subjects can contact should they have concerns.

Confidentiality of data

As with all clinical records, it is essential that the research subject's confidentiality is protected. In a research context this means ensuring that individual patients will not be identifiable from published research and that only appropriately authorised personnel have access to patients' records. Patient autonomy requires that patients ordinarily consent to anyone having access to their clinical records. This is especially important in research where the primary purpose is not to benefit the individual but to yield generalisable data which may be of benefit to future patients.

Richenda Power agues that the nature of a holistic consultation is such that notes are likely to include a lot of highly personal information about a person. Patients may object to their notes being used for research for this reason.[23] Moreover, many patients choose to consult a complementary practitioner precisely because they perceive that this is a more private experience than state-provided health care and so that they can discuss their problems freely and openly without fearing that there will be an official record which could be used without their knowledge for purposes other than treatment.

Determining acceptable levels of risk

In any research trial, the amount of harm to which a subject can be exposed must be the minimum compatible with achieving the desired outcomes. In other words, a risk/benefit calculation must ensure that subjects are not exposed to unreasonable levels of risk. More often than not, risk is usually understood in terms of physical harm to the research subject (although it is recognised that research on mentally incompetent groups should not be carried out if this would cause them undue emotional/psychological distress). The more holistic the therapy, the greater the risk that both treatment and research might lead to psychological and physiological harm. In assessing whether the level of risk is acceptable, the REC/review board will wish to satisfy itself as to the following:

- The research must be scientifically valid – the trial design must be capable of delivering the information sought.
- The investigator must be competent to conduct the research – this would include asking whether the lead researcher is sufficiently competent to manage the research project (often a very arbitrary and biassed assessment).
- The research must be necessary – research subjects should not be exposed to any level of risk, however small, if the research is unnecessary, in the sense that it is a duplication of research that has already been conducted or poses a question which it is not worth asking in the first place.

Making treatment more effective: incorporating research activities into practice

Many CAM therapists are daunted by the prospect of original research, but do not realise that there are other ways in which they could be systematically evaluate their practice. Therapists might like to consider the following activities, either independently, or in collaboration with colleagues:

- *Audit.* Unlike research, audit involves monitoring a practitioner's *processes* rather than outcomes and is a tool for ensuring quality service-provision. Unlike research, which seeks to ask questions of a generalisable nature, audit asks quite specific questions about various aspects of good patient care, for example, comprehensive history-taking, communication with a patient's GP, or following up patients who drop out of therapy. Audit is a threefold process which involves measuring one's practice (ideally against agreed professional standards), reflecting on areas where those standards are not met, and implementing changes in practice on the basis of these findings. An audit can be repeated to ensure that improvements are maintained. Auditing one's practice will improve efficiency but is not used to determine clinical effectiveness. It is widely regarded as an effective component of quality assurance and professional bodies are beginning to develop standards against which audits can be performed.
- *Outcome studies.* Any therapist who maintains effective, comprehensive notes ought to be able to conduct an outcome study. Unlike a trial, in which the researcher tests a hypothesis, an outcome study allows thera-

pists to monitor patients' progress, in terms of symptom-control, well-being and satisfaction, which are important aspects of practitioner development and can provide external benefit, for example, by increasing referral rates. Basic clinical questions might include:

- Does the treatment work?
- Do some patients get worse as a result of the treatment?
- If the treatment is successful, how long do the effects last?
- Which of a range of treatments is most effective?
- What qualities in the therapist affect the outcome?
- What expectations of the patient affect the outcome?

Practitioners might find it instructive to compare their outcomes with other practitioners who have used a same or different therapeutic approach to begin to think more systematically about what works in treatment. Various patient-centred outcome measures exist, such as the MYMOP questionnaire.[24] This may be an effective tool in ensuring that the outcomes measured reflect the measurements patients regard as important, which may, in turn, enhance the therapeutic relationship.

- *Case histories.* Although low down in the traditional hierarchy of evidence, therapists may find it beneficial to their practice to write up and share case studies with other colleagues. Although these reports will be anecdotal, they may be useful to the wider research community, particularly where the case is unusual. Therapists might consider writing these up and submitting them for publication in their professional journal as an aspect of continuing professional development (CPD).
- *Diagnostic reliability.* Another useful mechanism for ensuring consistency and reliability is for several practitioners to compare their diagnoses for several patients (with, of course, the patients' consent). Practitioners would not know what diagnosis their colleagues had made until all practitioners had diagnosed all patients. Correlating these results can improve practitioners' diagnostic skills and form the basis of future practitioner development/CPD activity.
- *Recording and reporting adverse effects.* Hopefully, most therapists will experience few serious adverse side effects in their practice. Where, however, an adverse event occurs, it will not contribute much to the overall knowledge base of the profession if the information is recorded only in the practitioner's personal files. Practitioners might contemplate writing up adverse events in a case study in their professional journal or newsletters, and professional bodies should be encouraged to maintain a regularly updated systematic database of adverse events, so that safety standards can be improved.

Notes

1 Cohen. M.H. (1998) *Complementary and Alternative Medicine. Legal Boundaries and Regulatory Perspectives.* Johns Hopkins University Press: Baltimore, MD and London.
2 Harman, W. and de Quincey, C. (1994) *The Scientific Explanation of Consciousness: Towards and Adequate Epistemology.* Institute of Noetic Science: Sausilito, CA. Cited in Cohen, op. cit.
3 Quality of life assessment is now a respected component of much health care research. See, for example, Muldoon, M., *et al.* (1998) 'What are Quality of Life Measurements Measuring?' *British Medical Journal.* 316: 542–545.
4 Fulder, S. (1988) 'The Basic Concepts of Alternative Medicine and Their Impact on Our Views of Health'. *The Journal of Alternative and Complementary Medicine.* 4(2): 147–158.
5 Cassidy, C.M. (1996) 'Cultural Context of Complementary and Alternative Medicine Systems'. In Micozzi, M. (eds) *Fundamentals of Complementary and Alternative Medicine.* Churchill Livingstone: Edinburgh.
6 Ibid.
7 Canter, D. and Nanke, L. (1993) 'Emerging Priorities in Complementary Medical Research'. In Lewith, G.L. and Aldridge, D. (eds) *Clinical Research Methodology for Complementary Therapists.* Hodder & Stoughton: Sevenoaks.
8 Sackett, D.L., Rosenberg, W.M.C., Gray, J.A.M., Harnes, R.B. and Richardson W.S. (1996) 'Evidence Based Medicine: What It Is and What It Isn't'. *British Medical Journal.* 312: 71–72.
9 Kerridge, I., Lowe, M. and Henry, D. (1998) 'Ethics and Evidence Based Medicine'. *British Medical Journal.* 316: 1151–1153.
10 Davidoff, F., Haynes, B., Sackett, D. and Smith, R. (1995) 'Evidence Based Medicine. A New Journal to Help Doctors Identify the Information they Need'. *British Medical Journal.* 310: 1085–1086.
11 Sackett, *et al.*, op. cit.
12 Greenhalgh, T. (1999) 'Narrative Based Medicine in an Evidence Based World'. *British Medical Journal.* 318: 323–325.
13 Hope, T. (1996) *Evidence-Based Patient Choice.* King's Fund: London.
14 Lewith, G., *et al.* (2000) 'Complementary Medicine Must Be Research Led and Evidence Based'. *British Medical Journal.* 320: 188.
15 Vincent, C. and Furnham, A. (1997) *Complementary Medicine, A Research Perspective.* John Wiley & Sons. Chichester: Chapter 8.
16 In 1997, the US National Institutes of Health (NIH) spent less than 0.1 per cent of its overall research budget of $12 million investigating CAM modalities. See Patel, V. (1988) 'Understanding the Integration of Alternative Modalities into an Emerging Health Care Model in the United States'. In Humber, J. and Almeder, R. (eds) *Alternative Medicine and Ethics.* Humana Press: Totowa, NJ.
17 Resch, K.I., Ernst, E. and Garrow, J. (2000) 'A Randomized Controlled Study of Reviewer Bias Against an Unconventional Therapy'. *Journal of the Royal Society of Medicine.* 93(4), April: 164–167.
18 See, for example, Anthony, H.M. (1993) 'Some Methodological Problems in the Assessment of Complementary Therapy'. In Lewith, G.L. and Aldridge, D. (eds) *Clinical Research Methodology for Complementary Therapists.* Hodder & Stoughton: Sevenoaks; Nahin, R.L. and Straus, S.E. (2001) 'Research into Complementary and Alternative Medicine: Problems and Potential'. *British Medical Journal.* 322: 161–164.
19 Vincent, C. and Furnham, A., op. cit.
20 Ibid.
21 Ibid.

22 Johannessen, H. (1996) 'Individualised Knowledge: Reflexologists, Biopaths and Kinesiologists in Denmark'. In Cant, S. and Sharma, U. (eds) *Complementary and Alternative Medicines. Knowledge in Practice*. Free Association Books Ltd: London.

23 Power, R. (1996) 'Considering Archival Research in One's Own Practice'. In Cant, S. and Sharma, U., op. cit.

24 See Paterson, C. (1996) 'Measuring Outcomes in Primary Care: A Patient Generated Measure, MYMOP, Compared with the SF-36 Health Survey'. *British Medical Journal*. 312: 1016–1020; Paterson, C. and Britten, N. (2000) 'In Pursuit of Patient-Centred Outcomes: A Qualitative Evaluation of the "Measure Yourself Medical Outcome Profile"'. *Journal of Health Service Research Policy*. 5(1), January: 27–36.

9

SUPERVISION

Key ethical issues
- Supervision as an aspect of competent practice
- Competencies required of a supervisor
- Overcoming resistance to supervision
- Negotiating the supervisory relationship
- Securing patient consent to supervision

Supervision is the formalised monitoring of a practitioner by another person, usually, but not always, a more experienced professional in the same field. The aim of supervision is to facilitate both professional and personal development. As such, supervision is an essential component of safe and competent practice, the benefits of which have long since been widely recognised within counselling and psychotherapy. In its *Ethical Framework for Good Practice in Counselling and Psychotherapy*, the British Association for Counselling and Psychotherapy imposes a general obligation on all counsellors, psychotherapists, supervisors and trainers to receive supervision.[1]

There are two quite distinct sorts of supervision. The first refers to the supervision of a newly qualified practitioner. Many professional bodies recognise that the period immediately after registering can be extremely daunting for a novice practitioner and therefore require a formalised period of supervised practice by a more experienced colleague. This form of supervision may be useful when a practitioner still lacks confidence in his or her technical competence. Some regulatory bodies will not grant full registration until practitioners have completed a period of supervised practice, during which period the practitioner has only conditional registration.

The second sort of supervision refers to ongoing supervision throughout a therapist's career. This may take a number of forms. As with post-qualification supervision, the supervisor might be a more experienced practitioner working within the same therapeutic discipline. Alternatively, some practitioners opt for peer supervision, where the supervisor can be either a colleague working within the same discipline, or a colleague working within a different modality. Supervision may be on a one-to-one basis or group-based. Issues a practitioner might bring to supervision include:

- boundary issues;
- whether the practitioner's desire for power is undermining the patient's ability to think for themselves thus creating dependency;
- whether the practitioner's therapeutic approach is working effectively, and if not, what other approaches could be employed;
- whether to refer the client, and if so, to whom;
- when and how to terminate the therapeutic relationship.

Competencies required of a supervisor

Since the process of supervision is designed to bolster the competence of the supervisee, it is axiomatic that the person providing the supervision is competent to act as a supervisor. Being a skilful practitioner does not guarantee that a practitioner will be an effective supervisor. Professional bodies need to consider providing guidance as to when a registered practitioner should be regarded as ready to act as a supervisor, and the criteria by which a person may be judged as capable of acting as a supervisor.

If supervision is to be effective, the supervisor must be able to confront the practitioner if he believes that the supervisee's handling of the case is misguided. This implies that the supervisor will have wide experience of therapeutic encounters and possess the strong interpersonal skills necessary for making constructive criticism. These skills will be enhanced if the supervisor also has necessary support, and supervisors should, in turn, receive regular supervision.

Supervisors may act in an educative, supportive and managerial role. In the following vignettes, MacPherson demonstrates how these functions supervision might present:

> A practitioner knows he has a new patient next week who is a consultant psychiatrist with motor neurone disease, He is extremely worried and agitated about getting the treatment right (educative and supportive).

> A practitioner wants to start his practice from home but has no sink in his treatment room. A sink is required by Environmental Health regulations, but he wants to start practising straight away, saying he can't afford a sink yet (managerial).

> A practitioner has recently separated from her partner and feels very vulnerable and generally over-emotional. She is not sure whether she

should stop practising temporarily even though she believes that the quality of care her patients receive from her is good (supportive and managerial).[2]

Part of effective supervision is learning how to reconcile potentially conflicting roles as a supervisor. This is especially important where the supervisor also has direct line management over a supervisee, since this can potentially inhibit the supervisory relationship and prevent a supervisee from revealing doubts and insecurities about his competence.

Based on his research into supervision within psychotherapy and psychoanalysis and his experience as a trainer of supervisors, Szecsody observes that 'pedagogical competence is neither emphasized nor acknowledged as a prerequisite for working as a supervisor'.[3] He has found that much of the research into supervision focusses on how supervisors teach at the expense of how supervisees learn. This highlights the need for professional bodies to consider both the supervision needs of their members and the training needs of supervisors.

Why is supervision so important?

Supervision is an important mechanism for ensuring patient safety. The isolated manner in which many practitioners work means that they may lack the day-to-day support, professional reassurance, mentoring, companionship, wisdom and humour of colleagues. Not all of these needs will necessarily be met through supervision, but supervision can certainly provide the professional support required to ensure that the therapist is not the sole arbiter of whether his or her conduct is ethical or professional. Unless the practitioner's regulatory body demands supervision as a condition of ongoing registration, the impetus to obtain supervision must come from the individual.

Practitioners' motivations for working in a healing profession are complex and not always entirely altruistic. MacPherson notes that clarifying these motives is a useful and perhaps necessary prerequisite for sustaining effectiveness as a practitioner. He acknowledges that practitioners may be motivated by a desire to feel good about themselves and posits that the greater the need for praise and appreciation, the more vulnerable practitioners become to blame and failure.[4] Understanding these internal processes is important if practitioners are not to become discouraged and disillusioned.

Supervision is also an important tool in recognising, and developing strategies to prevent, 'burnout'. The concept of burnout is familiar to those working in all helping professions. Pines *et al.* describe burnout as:

the result of constant or repeated emotional pressure associated with an intense involvement with people over long periods of time.

Such intense involvement is particularly prevalent in health, educa-tion and social service occupations, where professionals have a 'calling' to take care of other people's psychological, social and physical problems. Burnout is the painful realization that they no longer can help people in need, that they have nothing left in them to give.[5]

Supervision as part of lifelong learning

Hawkins and Shohet note that supervision flourishes in a culture committed to learning and development. Such a culture is:

> built on a belief system that a great deal of therapy is about creating the environment and relationships in which clients learn about themselves and their environment, in a way that leaves them with more options than they arrived with.[6]

The underlying notion is that therapists are better able to facilitate this potential for growth in others if they are constantly learning and developing as professionals themselves. What follows from this view of supervision is:

- learning and development are seen as continuous and lifelong processes, which have as much importance for senior practitioners as inexperi-enced practitioners;
- problem situations are seen as important opportunities for learning and development;
- supervision is part of the learning cycle. It is not there to provide quick solutions, but part of the reflective process which allows for the develop-ment, planning and implementation of new ideas.[7]

Resistance to supervision

There are several reasons why practitioners may feel reluctant to seek out supervision. One reasons is that many therapists are good at giving but are not good at receiving. To receive supervision might be seen as a tacit acknowledgement of neediness, or even weakness on the part of the thera-pist. New practitioners may ignore their own needs, focussing on the needs of their patients. Yet, denial of one's own needs will ultimately prove to be counter-productive. MacPherson warns:

> The more we deny our own needs, inevitably our needs will at some point reappear in a less than clear and useful way. We may, for example start finding ourselves drained by each therapeutic encounter. We may even start hating our patients and feel relieved

when they cancel. All of these symptoms may simply be a response to not knowing what our needs are: our needs for support, for encouragement, for validation, for guidance and for someone just to be there when there is nothing else to do.[8]

As with other aspects of life-long learning, therapists will invariably have to pay for supervision out of their own pocket. Newly qualified practitioners might not think that the expense is justified, particularly if supervision is not mandatory. Also, practitioners may mistakenly believe that there is only one form of supervision, or that there are rigid rules delineating the supervisor/supervisee relationship. This view is extremely misguided. The supervisory relationship is as diverse as the therapeutic relationship, and it is down to the individual therapist to negotiate or contract with the supervisor so that the relationship is able to meet the therapist's needs and expectations.

Negotiating the supervisory relationship

There is no single model of what supervision should look like. How supervision proceeds is a matter to be negotiated between supervisor and supervisee. As with the therapeutic encounter, the supervisee is expected to be an active participant in supervision. Accordingly, it is not just the supervisor, but also the supervisee, who has responsibilities. Proctor suggests that as a supervisee, a practitioner has a duty to:

- identify practice issues with which the practitioner needs help and to ask for help;
- become increasingly able to share freely;
- identify what responses are wanted from the supervisor;
- become more aware of organisational contracts which affect supervisor, client and supervisee;
- be open to feedback;
- monitor tendencies to justify, explain or defend;
- develop the ability to discriminate what feedback is useful.[9]

A supervisor's responsibilities include:

- ensuring a safe space for the supervisee to lay out practice issues as she sees fit;
- challenging practice which the supervisor believes to be unethical, unwise or incompetent (including intervening when the practitioner's management of a case is putting the supervisee's client or third parties at risk);
- challenging supervisees' personal or professional blindspots;

128

- allowing supervisees to reach their own solutions, without superimposing own views;
- having the skills and flexibility to provide a range of responses and approaches geared to the appropriate level of the supervisee.

Supervision as a tool in preventing professional abuse

Practitioners who are committed to receiving supervision should, in theory, at least, be less likely to abuse clients. The gulf between training and practice is such that particular issues, such as sexual attraction towards clients, is rarely taught to pre-registration students. In fact, if these issues are raised before the trainee practitioner has had much clinical experience with real patients, he or she is likely to resist discussion about professional abuse. Supervision provides the ideal opportunity for the therapist to discuss his feelings in this regard, hopefully stemming the transition from having feelings of attraction to acting upon them.

Securing the patient's consent to supervision

Therapists have an obligation to disclose to their clients and patients if they are receiving supervision. Specifically, patients have a right to know whether the specific details of their case will be discussed between the therapist and the supervisor and if so, what rights to confidentiality they may expect in these circumstances, and whether the supervisor has any therapeutic obligations towards them. In 1984, the American Psychologists Association's Committee on Science and Professional Ethics and Conduct (Ethics Committee) issued a formal statement emphasising that members should disclose to clients at the outset of the professional relationship their use, or intended use, of supervisors, and the general nature of the information regarding the case which will be disclosed to the supervisor.[10]

Patients are unlikely to take exception to a confidential discussion about their case if they realise that supervision is designed to improve and safeguard the therapeutic relationship. For this reason, the fact of supervision should be disclosed at the onset of therapy. A practitioner who does not disclose this information to a patient is breaching the relationship of trust which underpins the therapeutic encounter. Failure to disclose could constitute a breach of the practitioner's duty of confidentiality towards the patient and might be considered as professional misconduct by the therapist's professional body.

Notes

1 British Association for Counselling and Psychotherapy (2001) *Ethical Framework for Good Practice in Counselling and Psychotherapy*. British Association for Counselling and Psychotherapy: Rugby, Para 26

2 MacPherson, H. (1993) 'The Path to Mastery. A Role for Supervision'. *European Journal of Oriental Medicine*. 1(2): 6–11.
3 Szecsody, I. (1997) '(How) Is Learning Possible in Supervision?' In Martindale, B., Morner, M., Rodriguez, M. and Vidit, J. (eds) *Supervision and Its Vicissitudes*. Karnac Books: London.
4 MacPherson, op. cit.
5 Pines, A.M., Aronson, E. and Kafry, D. (1981) *Burnout: From Tedium to Growth*. Cited in Hawkins, P. and Shohet, R. (eds) (1989) *Supervision in the Helping Professions*. Open University Press: Milton Keynes.
6 Hawkins, P and Shohet, R., op. cit.
7 Kolb, D.A., Rubin, I.M. and McIntyre, J.M. (1971) *Organizational Psychology: An Experiential Approach*. Prentice Hall: New York.
8 MacPherson, op. cit.
9 Proctor, B. (1988) *Supervision: A Working Alliance*. Alexia Publications: St Leonard's-on-Sea.
10 For further discussion, see Pope, K.S. and Vasquez, M. (1998) *Ethics in Psychotherapy and Counseling. A Practical Guide* (2nd edition). Jossey-Bass: New York.

10

CONTINUING PROFESSIONAL DEVELOPMENT

Key ethical issues
* Defining CPD
* Formal and informal CPD mechanisms
* Particular problems in implementing CPD for CAM

What is continuing professional development?

Professionals derive their legitimacy from an expert knowledge base which sets them apart from lay people. They are sought out precisely because they are in possession of this expert knowledge. A significant proportion of this knowledge is technical knowledge, the acquisition of which is essential to performing the competencies involved in the given profession. Strict criteria are laid down as to what needs to be included in a professional education, where this education is to be provided, who is to provide the education, and how the training is to be assessed. Satisfactory completion of a professional education is usually marked by admittance to some form of register to denote that a certain standard has been achieved and that the person who has attained this standard has the requisite standards to practise.

However, being a health professional is clearly about more than just passing exams. Professional practice invariably involves not just knowledge, but an ability to translate knowledge into action, through the competent performance of a range of professional skills. In addition to professional knowledge and skills, a practitioner is also expected to acquire *professional attitudes*. Concepts of professional knowledge, skills and attitudes are not static, but are constantly evolving. No-one could seriously think that the professional training a practitioner received twenty years ago could provide all the information the practitioner needs for safe and competent practice until retirement. Shifts in cultural perception, and the use of new technologies, including the impact of information technology (IT), have an impact on professional knowledge, skills and attitudes, and professionals have an ethical duty to keep themselves up to date.

131

Because professionals are committed to providing the best possible service to their clients, they must be aware of changes within their field and be prepared to adapt their own practice in the light of new evidence as well as in the light of accumulated experience. This is central to the concept of *lifelong learning*. Skilled practitioners should be committed to embracing change. This involves a willingness to adopt and create innovative approaches to practice. A healer who originally trained and has practised independently for many years, is likely to have to acquire new skills to work in an integrated health setting, such as working within a multi-disciplinary team, keeping computerised records, and auditing her practice. Professional practice now requires professionals to continue to develop their competence and expertise over the course of their career.

The formalised way in which professional learning becomes a life-long process is through continuous professional development, usually referred to as CPD. CPD involves more than technical competencies. Whereas competence-based practice is externally driven and is about minimum standards for safe practice, CPD should be hopefully internally motivated, arising from the practitioner's desire for self-development. The UK government has recently introduced CPD throughout the NHS. The core principles it espouses could be applied to CAM CPD. CPD should be:

- purposeful and patient-centred;
- participative, that is, fully involving the individual and other relevant stakeholders;
- targeted at identified educational need;
- educationally effective;
- focussed on the development needs of clinical teams, across traditional professional and service boundaries;
- designed to build on previous knowledge, skills and experience;
- designed to enhance the skills of interpreting and applying knowledge based on research and development.[1]

Formal and informal approaches to continuing professional development

Current CPD models make use of both formal and informal approaches. Formal approaches include:

- post-qualification courses;
- degrees, higher degrees and research degree courses;
- work-based learning contracts;
- supervision;
- attendance at conferences and seminars;
- undertaking research;
- presenting research papers.

Of these, 'refresher courses' and conferences which give attendees continuing education 'points' are probably the most popular. Although conferences and courses are easy to accredit, they may lead to a superficial understanding of continuing professional development and not the deeper personal and professional development these activities are intended to stimulate.

Informal approaches to CPD include:

- independent study;
- reading journals and research papers;
- evaluating professional papers;
- keeping a professional diary or portfolio;
- reflecting on day-to-day practice;
- critical incident analysis;
- clinical reasoning.

What counts as CPD will vary from one therapy to another and one therapist to another. Whereas psychotherapists and counsellors may consider being in therapy themselves as a legitimate aspect of their ongoing professional development, practitioners of oriental therapies such as shiatsu and acupuncture could feel that training in Tai Chi or Qi Gong exerts a similar function. MacPherson argues that deeper approaches to CPD:

> recognise that personal development is often inextricably linked to one's development as a practitioner, that a shift in values can have a profound effect on the quality of one's practice and that a growing awareness of ethics, say, for example, becoming aware of our prejudices, could significantly influence the way our practice grows.[2]

Whether formal or informal approaches to CPD are undertaken, what is important is that these are reflected upon and feed back into professional practice. Experience from other health professions suggests that mandatory attendance of courses is useless unless steps are taken to feed the newly acquired knowledge into the workplace. Mere attendance is unlikely to affect practice. An obvious way to make CPD a higher priority to CAM practitioners is to tie it into ongoing professional registration.

Continuing professional development as an aspect of ongoing registration and revalidation

Increasingly, health care professionals are expected to be able to demonstrate their ongoing competence through revalidation or re-certification. It may be that thinking about formal systems of revalidation is premature in relation to CAM, when a proportion of CAM practitioners are not even required to demonstrate their initial competence to practise. Nonetheless, the issue of revalidation is an important one for newly emerging CAM professions to consider. If professional bodies are genuinely committed to protecting patients, they need to consider putting in place mechanisms which can measure that practitioners' skills are up to date and that practitioners are operating within the highest ethical standards. A professional disciplinary committee is unlikely to deal leniently with a practitioner who harms a patient through the use of outmoded, discredited techniques.

In terms of professional regulation, CPD is an integral part of the revalidation process. Re-certification or revalidation depends on the practitioner having undertaken a specified amount of training each year. In the UK, osteopaths and chiropractors have CPD requirements built into their statutory framework, although at the time of writing, no mandatory scheme is yet in place for these professions. Amongst the voluntary self-regulated professions, few therapies have formal systems of CPD in place, although in the UK initiatives are being implemented by professional bodies within homoeopathy, acupuncture and herbalism. The Society of Homoeopaths has introduced practice audit skills into homoeopathic education and is piloting linking this to professional registration. The National Federation of Spiritual Healers recognises the need for further CPD courses to be developed in healing, including specialised training for healers working with the medical profession in areas such as drug addiction, cancer and hospice care. The General Chiropractic Council supports the development of interdisciplinary CPD.[3]

The lack of statutory regulation in the UK makes it harder, but by no means impossible, to implement, or encourage, the development of CPD initiatives. Since practitioners are not required by law to belong to a professional registering body, the obvious means of enforcing CPD as a requirement for ongoing registration does not apply. Practitioners must therefore exercise self-responsibility in assessing their ongoing educational needs and undertaking CPD.

The commitment towards lifelong learning is explicit in the quality-orientated NHS. Whereas orthodox professionals will have contractual obligations and incentives to comply with CPD, for most CAM practitioners, the onus is on the individual practitioner to keep skills up to date and to monitor their own practice continuously. A recent government document in the UK demonstrated the commitment to CPD within the NHS. The centrality of CPD to clinical governance and quality assurance was emphasised, as was the need to set CPD in the context of partnerships between health professionals and their managers, employers and organisation. Many of the core principles of CPD identified have relevance to CAM.

Making continuing professional development relevant to CAM practitioners

Designing appropriate models for CPD within CAM must take account of the unique way in which CAM professionals work. Any such model must therefore acknowledge:

- most therapists work in sole practice rather than in organisations which are committed to CPD;
- few, if any, therapists will be funded for CPD activities, so will be paying for CPD out of their own pockets;
- CPD activities may need to take place in the evening or at weekends when practitioners are less likely to be seeing clients;
- not all therapists belong to a professional register, so accreditation of CPD cannot be linked solely to professional registration;
- many therapists may cross-specialise and belong to a number of professional organisations, so CPD activities need to be geared towards practitioner development and not just technical competence.

Is CPD necessary for all therapists?

The need for continuing professional development is unarguable. The UK government has supported the recommendations of a House of Lords Select Committee Report and wants all CAM regulatory bodies to promote life-long learning amongst their practitioners by setting standards of clinical practice and promoting effective systems of CPD.[4] The pace of social change and technological developments is such that modern health care practitioners need regular input to keep themselves up to date. The need to be aware of developments in medicine as a whole means that even therapists whose own therapeutic practice is less obviously technologically based still need to keep themselves up to date about advances in health care generally, as this may affect contraindications to treatment and influence referral decisions. In the absence of mandatory CPD, CAM therapists could usefully focus on practice-based activities such as in-depth case-history analysis, peer supervision, one-to-one supervision, self-directed learning about a difficult disease or condition and developing mentor relationships with more senior practitioners.[5]

Critically, the concept of CPD is about much more than the technical aspects of training, and is as concerned with a practitioner's personal and professional development. As pre-registration and undergraduate curricula become more and more crowded, some non-technical aspects of the therapeutic encounter (which a therapist should ideally have had at least some exposure to prior to setting up practice) will now be left to CPD providers. Issues which effective CPD might be concerned with include:

- reflective practice;
- updating technical competencies in light of the best available evidence;
- team-working, inter-disciplinary collaboration;
- research and audit skills and how to incorporate these into daily practice;
- management skills;
- ethical and legal aspects of practice.

Understanding reflective practice

Reflective practice involves thinking about both the positive and negative aspect of one's work, thinking critically about why things might have gone the way they did, asking whether, in retrospect, one would handle situations in a similar or different way in the future, and thinking about ways in which one might learn from past actions and introduce innovations into one's practice.

In the past, it was assumed that 'technical rationality' could provide solutions to all of the problems which presented themselves in a professional setting. Schön, whose work has been highly influential in this field, highlights that not all aspects of professional practice draw on technical expertise.[6] Problems arising in what Schön describes as the 'swampy lowlands of professional practice' may require alternative means of inquiry and resolution. Schön proposes one possible approach to reflective practice which has been widely applied in other health professions. Acknowledging the internalised process of thinking on one's feet, the *knowing-in-action* that most professionals demonstrate for dealing with situations, he nonetheless makes the point that when something out of the ordinary has happened, this requires a special type of consideration, which he calls '*reflection-in-action*'. He goes on to suggest that this process becomes useful when it is followed by '*reflection on reflection in practice*'. In this manner, practitioners actively learn from their actions and feed what they have learned into future encounters with patients.

An alternative model for reflecting on practice is that proposed by Kolb.[7] His focus is more on experiential learning. He distinguishes between learning through and learning from experience. His experiential learning model proposes a continuum of:

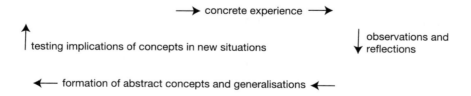

Whichever model is used, the message for practitioners is clear. Rather than proceeding through professional practice in an uncritical manner, treating each new situation and therapeutic encounter in isolation, therapists should strive to build on their previous experiences. This involves reflecting on both negative and positive aspects, and learning from them to improve one's future practice. This will not only enrich the therapist's practice but provide necessary safeguards for patients.

Peer review

Another useful tool in promoting good practice which can also be seen as an element of CPD is peer review. As its name suggests, peer review is a mechanism by which one's professional practice is observed by a peer who is able to offer feedback. Usually, although not necessarily, this will be someone who is trained in the same therapeutic discipline and who is roughly of the same experience (rather than someone who is noticeably more senior). Peer review is a voluntary and confidential process, which should be regarded as entirely separate from disciplinary mechanisms. Peer review requires honesty, openness and a sense of humour on the part of the reviewer and the person being reviewed. Feedback might include observations on the practitioner's choice of treatment, their communication style, including verbal and non-verbal communication, and the quality of record-keeping.

As with supervision, if the peer reviewer is to sit in on therapeutic encounters, this can only be done with the express consent of the client, who should be reassured that the peer reviewer is professionally trained and duty-bound to respect the patient's confidentiality. Often, therapists will choose who they wish to work with as a peer supervisor. If peer review is organised by a third party, for example, the therapists' training school, care must be taken to ensure that the practitioners do not have a personal or adverse relationships with the chosen peer and that the parties recognise the ethical obligations involved in peer review.

Political significance of CPD

There is no doubt that well organised CPD is a sign of a mature profession and is integral to maintaining high standards of professional practice. Most statutorily regulated professions now have CPD built in to their governing regulations as a condition of ongoing registration. Other voluntary self-regulating bodies are beginning to develop a more systematic approach to CPD for their members. This is astute not just in terms of promoting higher professional standards, but also politically, as a precursor to pursuing statutory regulation. Even if therapy is not aspiring to statutory regulation in the immediate future, when it does, practitioners will have to demonstrate evidence of good practice. Ongoing CPD and evidence of reflective practice will facilitate that process. As well as raising the profile of the individual therapies, the promotion of CPD is an essential precursor to integration. This is largely because CPD will drive research initiatives, which in turn will create wider acceptance and promote integration of CAM and orthodox medicine.

Notes

1   NHS Executive (1999) *Continuing Professional Development: Quality in the New NHS.* The Stationery Office: London.
2   MacPherson, H. (1995) 'Great Talents Ripen Late: Continuing Education in the Acupuncture Profession'. *European Journal of Oriental Medicine.* 1(6), Winter: 35–39.
3   See responses from these bodies contained in *House of Lords Select Committee on Science and Technology's Report on Complementary and Alternative Medicine. Written Evidence* (2000). HL Paper 48. The Stationery Office: London.
4   *Government's Response to the House of Lords Select Committee on Science and Technology's Report on Complementary and Alternative Medicine* (2001). The Stationery Office: London.
5   MacPherson, H. op. cit.
6   Schön, D. (1983) *The Reflective Practitioner. How Professionals Think in Action.* Avebury: Aldershot.
7   Kolb, D. (1984) *Experiential Learning.* Prentice Hall: New York.

11

MAINTAINING BOUNDARIES
AND PREVENTING ABUSE

Key ethical issues
- Differentiating professional relationships from personal relationships
- Establishing and maintaining appropriate boundaries
- Why boundary violations occur
- Practical strategies for avoiding abuse or allegations of abuse by patients

All therapeutic relationships are based on trust. This implies that the therapist has the patient's best interests at heart, that the therapist will not exploit the therapeutic relationship to satisfy his/her own ends, that the therapist will behave in an appropriate manner which is conducive to allow healing to take place, and that the therapist will refrain from any behaviour which could harm the patient. Not abusing the professional relationship is implicit in the duty of non-maleficence, that is, the duty to refrain from deliberately harming the patient. Much of the research in this area has been conducted in relation to patients injured by psychologists or psychotherapists. There is a consistently high incidence of sexual involvement with patients in each of these therapies. Pope and Vasquez have found that that the adverse consequences for patients can be extremely serious and fall into ten general categories. These include impaired ability to trust, emotional lability, suppressed rage, increased suicidal risk and cognitive dysfunction.[1]

The precise incidents of abuse in CAM are unknown as many clients are too distressed, ashamed or embarrassed to report what has happened to them. They may, additionally, be thwarted by the absence of a disciplinary body to whom they can complain. What is clear from charities working with abused patients, is that no single health profession or therapy has a monopoly on professional abuse. Cases of abuse have been reported against doctors, nurses, psychologists, osteopaths, reflexologists and most other health professions. Abusers are predominantly (although not exclusively) male, and the abused are predominantly (although not exclusively) female. Since CAM practitioners may well be treating patients who have been the subject of professional abuse, this topic is relevant to all therapists.

In a survey of clients using their services, the UK based charity, Prevention of Professional Abuse Network (POPAN), found that a staggering 80 per cent of clients abused by health professionals had been abused as children.[2] This reinforces a wealth of literature which shows that victims of sexual, physical or emotional abuse in childhood tend to be revictimised in later life.[3] Jehu explains that that this is likely to be due to child abuse victims' learned helplessness, unassertiveness, low self-esteem, excessive dependency, oversexualisation and dissociation. However, as Jehu makes clear:

> This psychological approach to explaining vulnerability in no way implies that patients are to blame for being abused by their therapists, who retain ethical responsibility for their actions.[4]

Although some experts feel that tighter regulatory controls will reduce the incidences of abuse, I have argued that whether a therapy is or is not statutorily regulated will not determine whether individual practitioners will act ethically. This is borne out by the fact that high incidences of abuse are being reported within statutory professions as well as within voluntarily regulated professions.

Aspects of CAM practice which render practitioners prone to abuse/abuse charges

Features unique to the CAM context mean that CAM practitioners need to be particularly sensitive to boundary issues. The following aspects of the CAM relationship can be problematic.

Setting

Although a number of therapists work from a clinic or other multi-practitioner setting, many practitioners work from a room in their own home. Although this is not inherently dangerous, it poses a number of problematic issues in terms of boundaries. Unless the therapist's treating room is accessed through a separate entrance, the therapist is automatically revealing a lot more about himself or herself than is the case in a clinical setting, and ordinarily therapists working from home should have a clearly delineated treatment area.

A shiatsu practitioner works from home in a tranquil setting. One hour into a two-hour treatment session, the telephone rings. The prac-

*titioner takes the call from his partner to discuss evening arrange-
ments. The practitioner speaks in code, in deference to his client's
presence, replying in monosyllables, interspersed with the occasional
and 'ditto', 'I do' and 'Me, too'. Although the call takes less than two
minutes, the client feels very put out by this intrusion and cannot relax
for the rest of the session, having been jolted into the realisation that
the practitioner has an outside life and is probably thinking more
about a romantic evening than the remainder of this treatment
session. The client thinks that it would be inappropriate to complain,
but comes away thinking rather less of the therapist than at the
outset.*

The absence of colleagues within earshot or the possibility of anyone to
disturb the consultation may have positive effects in that the patient feels
that she is genuinely receiving the therapist's quality time. However, the
isolation may also encourage professional abuse. Abusive practitioners have
been known to schedule appointments at the end of the working day or at
the weekend, when they are less likely to be disturbed.

Relaxed demeanour

Many (although not all) therapists either intuitively have, or deliberately
cultivate, a relaxed demeanour with their patients. For the main part, this is
a reflection of better communication skills and an ability to show the
empathy and genuine positive regard which encourages patients to open up
to the therapist. In the vast majority of cases, this manner is consistent with
effective clinical practice. Indeed, it is increasingly recognised that the non-
specific aspects of the therapeutic relationship may be of tremendous value.
Nonetheless, some patients may confuse the lack of formality on the part of
the therapist with a keenness to engage on a personal, rather than therapeutic, level. Indeed, many patients may feel genuinely confused by the
attention given to them by their therapist.

As in psychotherapeutic relationships, unconscious forces operate
between clients and their therapists. The notion of 'transference' describes
the way in which a patient's feelings and actions towards their therapist is
influenced by early childhood experiences, especially relationships with
parents. Therapists, in turn, exhibit counter-transference, their own unconscious fantasies and wishes about their patients. Practitioners need to be
aware of these forces and use them constructively in the professional relationship. This requires practitioners to have sufficient self-awareness and
detachment from their own responses to be able to understand the interaction between themselves and their patients.

Practitioners should never use patients as a means to an end, and should
not encourage a patient's undue dependence or idolisation of them.

Arguably, when the therapy involves physical contact, such as massage, osteopathy, chiropractic or shiatsu, the problems of misinterpretation are even more acute.

A woman with low self-esteem has derived considerable benefit from her relationship with her Qi Gong teacher. Since the teacher is of a similar age, and shares many of the same interests, she is surprised and upset when the teacher declines an invitation to come to her birthday party. Although she gives an excuse, the woman is convinced that her teacher does not like her and stops taking classes.

Patients' relative lack of knowledge

Many patients consulting a new therapist for the first time may genuinely not know what the therapy entails. Unless the patient has contacted a reputable professional organisation prior to the consultation, she is unlikely to know whether what the practitioner is doing is par for the course. Whereas popular culture gives most patients a reasonable idea of what is likely to happen to them when they have a medical consultation, patients may have very little idea of what a CAM consultation involves. Areas of confusion may include matters such as: whether it is standard to remain fully or partially dressed during the consultation; whether it is really necessary for the practitioner to remove underwear; whether intimate questions about the patient's anatomy and attitude towards sex are necessary for the diagnosis; whether it is appropriate for the practitioner to videotape the consultation; whether an intimate examination is therapeutically indicated; or whether the use of external relaxants, such as dimmed lights/candlelight, the burning of incense or relaxing aromatherapy oils or the playing of trance-inducing music are appropriate.

A patient has her first appointment with a masseur, who specialises in 'rolfing'. The patient knows very little about this particular form of massage other than its reputation as being very good at releasing deep muscle tension. The patient is prepared, at the therapist's recommendation, to undress fully, but becomes very uncomfortable when the therapist lies with his full body weight on her back, and is noticeably aroused. The patient says that this is not what she was expecting and terminates the session.

Erring on the side of caution, most codes of ethics are prescriptive, urging, for example, the presence of a chaperone during intimate examination. In terms of ethical guidance, a practitioner will be acting legitimately provided the intervention is based on explicit, informed consent, and the therapist believes that the treatment is in the patient's best interests, ideally on the basis of evidence.

Lack of formal regulation

In the UK, a significant proportion of practitioners do not belong to a regulatory body, eschewing the formalism and political implications they assume membership of a professional organisation brings. This presents additional concerns in terms of boundaries, in that the practitioner will not be working within any code of ethics, and in the event of the practitioner behaving unethically, the patient will not have a disciplinary mechanism or complaints procedure to rely upon. Practitioners who are minded to abuse may feel that they are more likely 'to get away with it' if they remain outside the reaches of professional associations. A prohibition in a code of ethics is scarcely likely to deter a practitioner from abusing. However, the knowledge that one's professional body operates a zero policy against professional abuse and encourages patient complaints may serve as a more effective deterrent.

> *In the above example, the patient, after discussing what happened with friends, resolves to initiate a complaint against the practitioner. Although the masseur claimed to be a member of a particular massage organisation, the patient is dismayed to discover that he has not been a registered member for several years. The organisation is sympathetic, but unable to help.*

Defining professional abuse

The nurses' and midwives' regulatory body in the UK, the UKCC, recently issued guidelines on professional abuse, defining it as follows:

> Abuse within the practitioner–client relationship is the result of the misuse of power or a betrayal of trust, respect or intimacy between the practitioner and the client, which the practitioner should know would cause physical or emotional harm to the client. Abuse takes many forms and may be physical, psychological, verbal, sexual, financial/material or based upon neglect.[5]

Sex with existing clients is the paradigmatic example of professional abuse, but the scope of abuse is much broader. Although these aspects of abuse may seem self-evident, it is worth setting out how the nurses' professional body, the UKCC, define these different manifestations of professional abuse: [6]

143

Physical abuse

Physical abuse is any physical contact which harms clients or is likely to cause them unnecessary and avoidable pain and distress. Examples include handling the client in a rough manner, giving medication inappropriately, poor application of manual handling techniques or unreasonable physical restraints. Physical abuse may cause psychological harm.

Psychological abuse

Psychological abuse is any verbal or non-verbal behaviour which demonstrates disrespect for the client and which could be emotionally or psychologically damaging. Examples include mocking, ignoring, coercing, threatening to cause physical harm or denying privacy.

Verbal abuse

Verbal abuse is any remark made to or about a client which may reasonably be perceived to be demeaning, disrespectful, humiliating, intimidating, racist, sexist, homophobic, ageist or blasphemous. Examples include making sarcastic remarks, using a condescending tone of voice or using excessive and unwanted familiarity.

Sexual abuse

Sexual abuse is forcing, inducing, or attempting to induce the client to engage in any form of sexual activity. This encompasses both physical behaviour and remarks of a sexual nature made towards the client. Examples include touching a client inappropriately or engaging in sexual discussions which have no relevance to the client's care.

Financial/material abuse

Financial/material abuse involves not only illegal acts such as stealing a client's money or property but also the inappropriate use of a client's funds, property or resources. Examples include borrowing property or money from a client or a client's family member, inappropriate withholding of a client's money or possessions and the inappropriate handling of, or accounting for, a client's money or possessions.

Neglect

Neglect is the refusal or failure on the part of the registered nurse, midwife or health visitor to meet the essential care needs of a client. Examples include failure to attend to the personal hygiene of a client, failure to communicate adequately with the client and the inappropriate withholding of food, fluids, clothing, medication, medical aides assistance or equipment.

Exploring how professional relationships differ from personal relationships

Perhaps the most appropriate starting point of any discussion on professional abuse is identifying what differentiates a professional relationship from a personal relationship. Although the characteristics of a professional relationship are rarely spelt out, duties of professionals might include the following:

- maintaining appropriate physical boundaries;
- avoiding sexual relationships with patients/clients;
- not allowing patients to become unduly dependent;
- not having preferences – treating all patients equally, respecting their value as individuals and not having favourites;
- not displaying anger or irritation and never using violence or force other than in self-defence;
- refraining from excessive personal disclosure and not burdening clients/patients with personal problems;
- maintaining a level of formality and distance.

Customarily, professionals give and patients take, in exchange for a fee. Whereas professional relationships are limited in time and space, personal relationships may develop and be sustained over a lifetime. Personal relationships are usually marked by some or all of the following:

- liberty to choose friends/partners;
- preferences are natural and desirable;
- emotional and physical intimacy;
- love;
- equality between the parties;
- interdependence/leaning on each other;
- mutual responsibility/give and take;
- shared values and interests;
- ability to display anger or to be rude.

Doubtless, many other characteristics could be added to each list. Essentially, the object of this exercise is to demonstrate that even if the differences are hard to articulate, personal relationships and professional relationships are not the same thing and need to be kept separate in both the practitioner's mind and the patient's mind. There are, however, a number of similarities and areas of overlap between personal and professional relationships which may blur the distinction between what is and what is not acceptable behaviour. Consider the following examples:

- A sympathetic practitioner might easily respond to a patient's distress by putting a comforting arm around them.

- Whilst traditionally, health professionals give and patients take, many therapists consider themselves to be enriched by their clients.
- Some patients and therapists 'click' and the therapeutic relationship is strengthened by a sense of genuine empathy.
- A patient may share the practitioner's interests and values, and would be someone whose friendship the practitioner would cultivate in different circumstances.
- Some people don't like giving very much of themselves away or talking about their problems even to their closest friends.
- Some practitioners use an element of personal disclosure to reassure the patient and to gain their trust.
- Although it is often assumed that most personal relationships are based on a balance of power, many personal and sexual relationships are extremely one-sided, with one party being excessively controlling and the other highly dependent.

Far from being clear, these examples show that it may be less easy to demarcate professional relationships from personal relationships than first thought. The failure to address this issue early on in training may have disastrous consequences. A practitioner who is naturally short tempered, controlling, flirtatious or compassionate does not become a saint simply because he or she is acting in a professional capacity. Personal characteristics will not necessarily disappear simply because of the context of the encounter. Learning what is and is not appropriate behaviour is as much a part of professional training as acquiring professional skills. This requires explicit training for CAM practitioners on maintaining and establishing appropriate boundaries.

Establishing and maintaining appropriate boundaries

Establishing and maintaining appropriate boundaries is central to preventing professional abuse. Although the idea of boundaries is well explored in the psychotherapy literature, its relevance to the training and practice of CAM therapists has not been fully appreciated. Boundaries are important in any trust relationship, particularly in the healer/patient relationship where there is usually a power disequilibrium between the two parties. Whilst accepting that not all patients are vulnerable to abuse, it can be argued that any patient who is consulting a therapist for health reasons (as opposed to relaxation/leisure purposes) is in a relationship of reliance and need. This is likely to be exacerbated when the therapist is working with the patient on a psychological level, and not just a physical level, as will be the case with many CAM therapists.

Much pioneering work in the training and rehabilitation of abusing practitioners has been carried out by Gary Schoener. Schoener's work has contradicted many of the previously held assumptions about practitioners who abuse. He has found that whilst a proportion of sex offences is perpetrated by sexual predators and compulsive sex offenders, many abusing practitioners do not fall into these categories. Schoener similarly disputes that there is a clear and generally accepted definition of sexual misconduct, and this makes it particularly problematic to draw a line between those therapists whose behaviour could be rehabilitated and those who should be permanently removed from practice. He asks:

> Does a single inappropriate hug which has some erotic elements which is followed by an apology from the professional and appropriate consultation meet the criterion for expulsion from the field? What about inappropriate sexual comments? How much resolved erotic transference and seductive talk before the line is crossed?[7]

What emerges is the idea that all practitioners are open to boundary violation in certain circumstances. In terms of categorising situations in which therapists abuse, Schoener synthesises the findings of Pope and Bouhoutsos to describe the ten most common scenarios of psychotherapists' sexual misconduct.

Role trading: therapist becomes the patient.

Sex therapy: sex fraudulently presented as 'sex therapy'.

'As if': therapist ignores that feelings are likely to be transference.

Svengali: therapist exploits dependent client.

Drugs and/or alcohol: used in seduction.

Rape: overt force or threats are used by the therapist.

True love: therapist rationalises that it is 'true love'.

It just got out of hand: loss of control due to the emotional closeness of therapy.

Time out: therapist rationalises that contact outside of session is legitimate.

Hold me: in which the therapist exploits the patient's need to be held or touched.

Minimising the risk of boundary violations

One would hope that most therapists have sufficient propriety not to abuse their patients. Pope and Vasquez ask why the majority of practitioners do not abuse their patients.[8] The results of their study were revealing. Reasons given by social workers and psychologists for refraining from abuse included that sexual involvement with a patient would be: unethical, counter-therapeutic/exploitative, unprofessional, against the therapist's personal values, that the therapist was already in a committed relationship and that such a relationship could lead to censure or damage to reputation.

Such abuses are so inimical to the fundamental purpose of therapy that one might argue that prohibitions against abuse are too obvious even to include in codes of ethics. Sadly, the proportion of practitioners who abuse suggest that this is not the case, and prohibitions against practitioner/patient sexual contact have existed since at least Hippocratic times. Pope and Vasquez hypothesise:

> [T]hat the fact that this prohibition has remained constant over so long a time and throughout so many diverse cultures reflects to some extent the recognition that such intimacies place the patient at risk for exceptional harm.[9]

Avoiding professional abuse or accusations of professional abuse

The issue of abuse should be taken seriously by all working practitioners, since in these increasingly litigious times, therapists may also find themselves on the receiving end of a frivolous/malicious allegation, which could have devastating implications for a therapist's practice. Although it may be extremely difficult to curtail the activities of a serial abuser, there are several practical steps which therapists can take to minimise the likelihood of abusing, *or being accused of abuse*. These might include:

- Avoid inappropriate physical contact. Be sensitive to how patient will interpret physical contact. Some patients may welcome a reassuring hug at the end of a session, whereas other patients may regard this as highly intrusive.
- Avoid excessive self-disclosure. This may represent the start of a slippery slope in which the role of therapist and patient are reversed.
- Avoid personal intervention in a patient's personal problems (for example, lending money/helping patient find employment). These are likely to be counter-therapeutic in the long term, since they diminish the patient's ability to take self-responsibility and to act autonomously.
- Encourage patients to seek a second opinion or consult other therapists. Discouraging a patient from seeing other therapists may indicate a desire to exercise undue control over the patient and may suggest a wholly inappropriate dependence on the patient on the part of the therapist.
- Recognise the strength of counter-transference and take appropriate steps to deal with this. Specifically, practitioners should acknowledge their sexual attraction towards patients (which is not in itself unethical

and is widespread) and deal with this appropriately, for example, by consulting with colleagues or a supervisor or undertaking psycho-therapy.

- Have an awareness of cultural dimensions of appropriate boundaries. Patients may have widely varying cultural expectations of what is or is not appropriate in terms of physical contact and emotional engagement with a therapist. Therapists must act in a culturally acceptable fashion.
- Make use of chaperones when carrying out intimate examinations. This is a sensible precaution for the therapist's protection as well as the patient's.
- Ensuring that a physical examination which may involve the genital area is only carried out with the patient's written consent, which is documented in the patient's record.
- Work with a supervisor, and bring up uncomfortable issues in supervision, rather than keeping them inside. Wanting to keep aspects of patient relationships a secret may indicate that the therapist is acting furtively.

Miscellaneous concerns

Are sexual relationships with clients ever permissible?

Are sexual relationships ever permissible between therapists and patients whilst treatment is ongoing? The overwhelming consensus is that this is potentially extremely harmful to the patient. Jehu lists the following reasons for proscribing sexual activity:

- breach of trust;
- violation of the role of therapist;
- exploitation of vulnerability;
- misuse of power;
- absence of consent;
- impairment of the therapeutic process;
- iatrogenic effects;
- bringing the profession into disrepute.[10]

Although the position is less categoric in relation to former patients, there are still strong reasons why sexual relationships are to be avoided. If a practitioner and patient both consensually decide to pursue a sexual relationship, the therapeutic relationship must be terminated immediately and the therapist should refer the patient to a practitioner who can meet his or her therapeutic needs. Some professional organisations place a time limit on entering into a sexual relationship with a former client. The American

Counseling Association's 1996 Code of Ethics advises its members not to counsel persons with whom they have had a sexual relationship. As regards former clients, the Association advises:

> Counselors do not engage in sexual intimacies with former clients within a minimum of two years after terminating the counseling relationship. Counselors who engage in such a relationship after two years following termination have the responsibility to examine and document thoroughly that such relations did not have an exploitative nature, based on factors such as duration of counseling, amount of time since counseling, termination circumstances, client's personal history and mental status, adverse impact on the client, and actions by the counselor suggesting a plan to initiate a sexual relationship with the client after termination.

Practitioners should be aware that their professional bodies may also consider post-termination relationships to be unethical, depending on the facts of the individual case.

Difficulties for patients in initiating a complaint

For some patients, the prospect of bringing a formal complaint against a practitioner is a daunting task. Particularly in situations where there are no witnesses to the alleged abuse, the patient will be aware that any allegation will be the patient's word against that of the practitioner. The problem is compounded by the fact that a number of patients who are abused in therapeutic relationships are already victims of childhood sexual abuse. The likelihood of patients succeeding in bringing a criminal prosecution is hampered by patients' mental state and the fact that they may well have been presenting with depressive illness or emotional distress, which could render their evidence less reliable in a court of law. Professional bodies must make concerted efforts to ensure such complaints are heard and victims of professional abuse are supported.

Abuse against trainee practitioners

The same disequilibrium of power which facilitates abuse of patients extends to supervisors and their trainees. Boundary violations and professional abuse are also a problem for students of CAM therapies. Trainees may feel particularly disempowered from initiating a complaint for fear of failing the course, particularly when they are close to completing their studies. This is an area in which training schools and professional associations should be considering urgent action.

Financial abuse

Some practitioners may be genuinely surprised to see financial abuse listed in the same category as sexual abuse. Whilst the effects of the latter on the patient may be more devastating than the effects of financial abuse, both represent a fundamental abuse of the professional relationship and the trust placed in the practitioner by the client. It is hard to define the point at which overcharging should be described as abuse. Clearly, there is a variation in how much CAM practitioners charge, as indeed there is variation in how much clients are willing to pay. Higher fees do not necessarily correspond to a better quality of care or better treatment outcomes.

The absence of hierarchical structures within most therapies means that a recently qualified practitioner may decide to charge as much for their services as a more established practitioner. In this absence of professional guidelines, practitioners must determine for themselves how much their services are worth. The American Chiropractors Association's Code of Ethics states:

> Doctors of chiropractic are entitled to receive proper and reasonable compensation for their professional services commensurate with the value of the services they have rendered taking into consideration their experience, time required, reputation and the nature of the condition involved.

Financial abuse also occurs when a practitioner prolongs the professional relationship, even though the patient is no longer benefiting from it. The Chiropractors' Code continues:

> Doctors of chiropractic should terminate a professional relationship when it becomes reasonably clear that the patient is not benefiting from it.

This will always be a matter of judgement, and the preventative role of most therapies could see therapists offering treatment on a fairly open-ended basis. As in all areas, the practitioner should be motivated by what is in the patient's best interests.

Notes

1 Pope, K.S. and Vasquez, M. (1998) *Ethics in Psychotherapy and Counseling. A Practical Guide* (2nd edition). Jossey-Bass: New York.
2 Prevention of Professional Abuse Network (1999) *Annual Report*. POPAN: London.
3 See, for example, Pope, K.S. and Vetter, V.A. (1991) 'Prior Therapist–Patient Sexual Involvement Among Patients Seen By Psychologists'. *Psychotherapy*. 28: 429–438; Kluft, R.P. (1990) 'Incest and Subsequent Revictimization: The Case of

Therapist–Patient Sexual Exploitation, with a Description of the Sitting Duck Syndrome'. In Kluft, R.P. (ed.) *Incest Related Syndromes of Adult Psychopathology*. American Psychiatric Press: Washington, DC.
4 Jehu, D. (1994) *Patients as Victims, Sexual Abuse in Psychotherapy and Counselling*. John Wiley & Sons: Chichester.
5 United Kingdom Central Council for Nursing, Midwifery and Health Visiting (1999) *Practitioner–Client Relationships and the Prevention of Abuse*. UKCC: London.
6 Ibid., paras 13–18.
7 See, especially, Schoener, G. (1988) 'Assessment and Rehabilitation of Professionals Who Violate Sexual Boundaries With Clients'. In *Collected Papers on Professional Misconduct*. Good Faith & Associates: North Melbourne, Victoria, Australia.
8 Pope and Vasquez, op. cit.
9 Ibid.
10 Jehu, op. cit.

12

RESPECT FOR AUTONOMY
AND CONSENT

Key ethical issues
- Respect for autonomy and how this differs from patient-centred practice
- Understanding the legal requirements of consent
- Autonomy and consent issues specific to CAM practice

All codes of ethics stress the importance of respecting the patient autonomy. The principle of respect for autonomy requires that practitioners provide their patients with sufficient information to make informed choices and that practitioners respect the treatment choices patients make. The increased prominence of the duty to respect patient autonomy has had a profound influence on the health care relationships. Whereas Hippocratic and other ancient healing traditions have always stressed the duty of the physician to care for and benefit the sick, modern health carers are encouraged to treat patients as equal partners in a joint therapeutic alliance. This requires competent patients to take a full and active role in decisions regarding their treatment, although, in reality, the choices patients are offered have usually been predetermined by what the practitioner thinks is appropriate. The participatory model of autonomy also overlooks the extent to which illness may compromise a patient's autonomy and create a sense of dependence on the practitioner.

Nevertheless, the right to be consulted is now enshrined in law through the need to obtain a valid consent to treatment. Health carers who fail to provide patients with adequate information or treat patients against their wishes may be sued for negligence or trespass, even if they are acting in what they perceive to be the patient's best interests.

Despite an approach to healing which is avowedly patient-centred, it is not immediately obvious how much stronger the commitment to patient autonomy is within CAM. Whilst CAM practitioners tend to tailor their treatment to the individual, and provide ample time to listen to patients, the extent to which the patient is an active participant in that process may be quite minimal. Very few practitioners provide patients with written information about the risks involved in therapy or give patients time to decide whether they wish to go ahead or refuse treatment. In terms of written consent, most CAM practitioners assume that the mere fact the patient has come to consult them means that they impliedly agree to let the practitioner do whatever is felt to be in their best interests.

If this *is* an accurate reflection of how some CAM practitioners work, it raises profound questions about the role and scope of respect for autonomy and consent in CAM. What may emerge is that the fundamental differences identified between CAM and conventional health care may require a different understanding of respect for autonomy. The ramifications of this discussion are significant, since even if CAM therapists view autonomy differently to other health care practitioners, they still have a duty to work within the law, and may be sued if they do not obtain consent. If the current definitions of consent do not provide a helpful or applicable model to CAM, other mechanisms need to be put in place to ensure that the therapeutic encounter is congruent with the patient's expectations and values.

Does patient-centredness equate to respecting autonomy?

If anything, patients seem to consult CAM practitioners because they are perceived as being less paternalistic than doctors and more patient-centred. There may be very tangible reasons why patients feel that CAM therapists are more respectful of their autonomy. These include:

- CAM therapists have time to listen. The average consultation with a CAM practitioner may be between half an hour to an hour. This is considerably longer than the time patients get to spend with doctors (in the UK, the consultation time with general practitioners is less than ten minutes).
- CAM therapists appear to offer patients tailor-made treatment. Patients receiving product-based therapies are more likely to feel that they have been given a treatment suited to their individual circumstances than patients who are handed a prescription for penicillin.
- CAM therapists working holistically are likely to utilise Rogerian skills, including warmth, genuineness and empathy, and may have better communication skills than allopathic practitioners.

At the heart of CAM patient-centredness seems to be an attempt to put the patient's interpretation of their own illness and their aspirations at the centre of the therapeutic encounter. This is particularly important when patients suffer from chronic conditions. As Holm observes:

[C]hronic diseases involve the patient in a quite different way. The patients quickly learn the specific features of the disease as it manifests themselves in them. And whereas the doctor may be an expert on the disease in general, the patient soon becomes the foremost expert on *her* disease and its specific manifestations.[1] (original emphasis)

Patient-centredness, as understood by most practitioners, may have as much to do with the ethical duty to benefit patients as it does with respecting autonomy. All practitioners, be they conventionally trained or otherwise, need to develop the skills to determine what the illness means for this individual patient and how it affects their life in the context of their personal values. Health professionals are increasingly patient/client-centred, and conventional health care professionals may resent the accusation that they are not patient-centred. In an article exploring patients' motivations for seeking CAM, Vickers and Zollman comment:

All healthcare practitioners, conventional or complementary, aim to tailor their interventions to the needs of individual patients. However, conventional practitioners generally direct treatment at the underlying disease processes, whereas many complementary practitioners base treatment more on the way patients experience and manifest their disease, including their psychology and response to illness. Treatment is 'individualised' in both cases, but patients' personalities and emotions may be more influential in the latter approach.

What is clear is that the time that CAM practitioners spend with patients relative to the time spent with patients by doctors gives patients the opportunity to *feel* that they are being heard. Vickers and Zollman continue:

Although good conventional care involves considering the patient as a person, not a disease, time pressures can lead to an apparent emphasis on the physical aspects of illness. Some patients cite the lack of personal attention paid by conventional practitioners as a reason for choosing a complementary approach.[2]

Nonetheless, respect for autonomy involves more than just listening to patients, and a practitioner's warmth and empathy is no substitute for technical competence. Autonomy requirements go beyond seeking permission to treat. Respecting patient autonomy places positive obligations on health carers to facilitate patient choice. This involves spending sufficient time with patients to make sure they have sufficient information, in language they can understand, to help them reach the right choice for themselves. This includes a candid discussion of the options available to the patient and their relative costs and benefits. Viewed in this light, respecting autonomy is an ongoing process between the practitioner and patient and not a one-off event at the start of a therapeutic relationship. Respecting autonomy involves:

- consulting with the patient over all significant decisions, providing adequate information to facilitate patient choice, including the patient's absolute right to refuse treatment or choose a different practitioner;
- respecting patients' wishes;
- respecting patients' cultural and religious values;
- not exerting undue influence on a patient, for example, by categorically insisting the patient accepts the practitioner's view of the cause of the patient's illness;
- telling the truth;
- respecting the patient's privacy;
- respecting the patient's dignity;
- respecting the patient's confidentiality;
- respecting the autonomy of patients with limited capacity as far as is possible, whilst at the same time trying to protect them from making harmful choices.

The relationship between respect for autonomy and consent

The principle of respect for autonomy is supported by a legal duty to obtain the patient's consent. The purpose of obtaining consent is to ensure that the patient is making an informed, voluntary choice. In order to make legally valid choices, patients must have sufficient mental competence to understand the information they are given. The presumption is that adults have the capacity to make their own decisions. This does not mean that they have to be able to understand all the information they are presented with perfectly (a state of full autonomy), but that they have sufficient ability to make decisions which are congruent with their wishes and values (a state of substantive autonomy). There are two main reasons why consent is sought:

- to facilitate patient choice by giving the patient enough information to decide whether or not to accept the treatment;
- to avoid being sued for something going wrong which the patient was not warned about (negligence) or if the patient complains that they were treated against their wishes (battery).

From an ethical perspective, avoiding being sued is not an adequate or appropriate justification for seeking to obtain consent. Rather, consent is the mechanism through which the patient's autonomy can be respected. Patients cannot be truly autonomous and make the decisions which are right for them unless they have enough information to do so, and practitioners are prepared to accept their informed refusal of treatment as well as their agreement.

Obtaining consent is a *process*, rather than a single activity, designed to ensure that a patient continues to agree to the treatment which is being given. Although consent usually takes the form of a written consent form, consent can be verbal, depending on the circumstances. A form is only evidence to suggest that the process of obtaining consent has been followed through. An acupuncturist may ask the patient to sign a written consent form at the start of treatment. At each session, verbal consent should suffice, even if a new point is needled, but specific consent should be sought if the acupuncturist is about to use moxibustion (burning of herbs) for the first time. An osteopath may have secured the patient's consent to osteopathic treatment, but should seek additional consent if he intends to make use of acupuncture within a treatment session.

What does obtaining consent require?

There are three elements to obtaining a valid consent:

- patients must be given adequate information;
- patients must be competent to consent;
- the patient's decision must be voluntary.

How much information must be given?

This must be determined in accordance with the prevailing standard of care in the therapy at the particular point in time. Broadly speaking, patients must be told of any risks which a reasonable practitioner would give and any risks that a reasonable patient would regard as material to their decision-making. This will include probable risks as well as less likely, but more serious, risks. Practitioners should answer any direct questions fully and truthfully.

> *An aromatherapist fails to tell a patient that she should not go in the sun directly after her treatment, as the citrus oils which she has just used will make the patient's skin photosensitive. The patient spends the rest of the day sunbathing on the beach and suffers bad burns.*

> *An acupuncturist is running late and forgets to tell a new client that he may feel light headed for a short while after the treatment and should rest in the waiting room until he feels steady. Unfortunately, the patient gets straight into his car and causes a collision.*

In each case, the practitioner has failed to provide information which has resulted in harm to the patient. Whether these patients could successfully sue for negligence depends on what warning a reasonable practitioner would have given. In each case, the patient might also have been expected to exercise self-responsibility and if sued, the practitioners might be able to claim that there was contributory negligence on the patient's part.

A patient only needs to be told about risks which are inherent in therapy. Although an incompetent acupuncturist may cause a patient a pneumothorax, this should not happen if the acupuncturist is competent. Accordingly, this is not a risk that needs to be disclosed.

Patient must be competent

This means that the patient must be capable of weighing up the information given and using it to arrive at a rational choice. Competence is decision-specific, so that a patient may be deemed competent to take some decisions but not others. Adults are presumed to be competent to make their own health care decisions.

> *A massage therapist is employed by a psychiatric unit specialising in eating disorders. Before providing a treatment, the therapist needs to ensure that her patients are mentally competent to agree to treatment, since the nature of their illness may distort their ability to arrive at a rational decision.*

> *A reflexologist is employed to treat patients in a residential unit for adolescents with learning disabilities. Although her patients lack the mental capacity to make many complex decisions, she judges them competent to agree to treatment.*

To be competent to consent, patients only need to understand in broad terms what is involved in the treatment. Most CAM consultations involve competent adults who have chosen to seek out therapy. A practitioner may feel that a patient is not competent to consent to a particular session, for example, if they turn up for a session after drinking or taking drugs. If the practitioner decides that a patient, for whatever reason, is not competent to consent, then the practitioner can only give treatment which is in the patient's best interests.

> *A healer is asked by a patient's family to treat their relative, who is in a coma. Having secured permission from the clinician in charge, the healer decides that it is appropriate to provide treatment.*

Voluntariness of the decision

The patient's decision must be voluntary. The patient should not be subject to undue coercion, for example by the therapist, or by a member of their family, urging them to accept treatment against their wishes. In order to make the consent process meaningful, patients must feel they are able to reject as well as accept treatment proposals.

Over a period of weeks, a timid patient is persuaded by her domineering therapist to undergo a 'rebirthing' experience. Unfortunately, the session triggers potent and painful memories for the patient, who is extremely distressed and does not return for further treatment.

A man presents for psychotherapy saying that his wife has sent him. The man insists that there is nothing wrong with him and that it is his wife who needs therapy. The psychotherapist finds the patient to be rational and lucid and tells the patient that unless he actively wants to engage in the psychotherapeutic process, there is little that the therapist can do for him.

Practitioners should bear in mind that illness may deprive patients of some of their autonomy and that this may render some patients unusually suggestible. Since practitioners can assume tremendous significance in their patient's lives, they should be careful not to impose their own views about what is good for the patient. As the second case demonstrates, in most CAM encounters it will be difficult to proceed unless the patient voluntarily accepts treatment.

Centrality of consent to CAM practice

The legal duty to obtain consent is as relevant to CAM practice as it is conventional medicine. Yet, many CAM therapists across a range of disciplines think that the subject of informed consent has little relevance to them. Several reasons might be advanced:

- Many therapists may feel that if the client has voluntarily sought out the therapist, then consent can be implied.
- In the absence of any ethical or legal content in their training, some therapists may not really understand what obtaining consent involves or that there are legal implications for failing to obtain consent.
- Some therapists may mistakenly think that consent is only relevant where the procedure poses serious physical risks of harm to a patient.
- Some therapists may mistakenly think that consent is only relevant where the procedure involves physical touching.
- Some therapists assume that formal consent mechanisms are only necessary in a medical culture where patients sue, that is, in conventional medicine.

- Some therapists actively reject the notion that the patient should be given information and asked to make a choice. Rather, they embrace paternalism as an active choice, feeling that this is most likely to benefit the patient.

These responses are not likely to stand up to legal scrutiny. All health care practitioners, including CAM practitioners, need to obtain consent to treatment. This includes providing information about side effects. The fact that the therapy may involve fewer side effects than say surgery, does not absolve the practitioner of the need to explain what the therapy is intended to do, what will be involved for the patient, what the patient can expect to feel like after the treatment, and what alternatives there are to what is being proposed. Failure to do so may have serious legal ramifications for the therapist and may seriously compromise the patient's trust and ability to make an informed choice. Although there has not been much litigation against CAM therapists to date, this may change as therapists become more visible and become integrated within conventional medical settings.

Practical suggestions for implementing consent

Many CAM practitioners already comply with consent requirements as an integral part of good practice and good communication. There are ways in which practitioners could formalise this process to ensure that there is no misunderstanding between them and their patients which could give rise to legal action or a professional complaint. Critically, CAM therapists should not assume that patients understand what their therapy involves. When patients make their first appointment, the therapist should either give them a leaflet there and then, or better still, send it to them in advance of the first session. This leaflet could usefully outline:

- what the therapy involves, that is, what will happen to the patient;
- how will the patient feel after the treatment, for example, will they be able to drive home?;
- the basic underlying philosophy of the therapy;
- how long the session is likely to last;
- how many sessions are likely to be necessary to bring about a material change in the patient's condition;
- what qualifications the practitioner has, and any particular areas of interest or expertise the practitioner has.

Additionally, practitioners might consider an initial session in which some of these issues are discussed in the light of the patient's particular circumstances, so that practitioner and patient can decide whether the particular approach is appropriate. These themes will be taken up in the section on negotiating contracts.

Theoretical difficulties of applying consent principles to CAM

Most practitioners recognise that obtaining consent is an important part of professional health care practice. CAM training schools are beginning to discuss ethical and legal requirements within their curriculum and many practitioners have devised systems for satisfying consent requirements. There are, nonetheless, some theoretical difficulties in applying conventional consent principles to some CAM relationships. These difficulties are not insurmountable, but merit further analysis.

Informational requirements

The most common problem in obtaining consent is perceived to be the lack of information known about many CAM therapies. It has been argued that in the absence of data from systematic research CAM practitioners are unable to give patients the information they need about the risks of treatment to enable them to make an informed choice. This argument falls into the trap of treating consent as a defence against being sued rather than viewing consent as a function and requirement of autonomy. Patients should not be expected to make better choices about their health than they do about other decisions in their lives. People ought to be allowed to decide for themselves how much information they feel they need to make a choice. If a patient is content to pursue a CAM therapy on the basis of the current available information, this is consistent with respecting their autonomy and consent can be obtained on the basis of the best available evidence. This does not mean that CAM practitioners do not have an ethical duty to work towards discovering information about risks, based on their ethical commitment to benefiting and not causing harm.

Provided the emphasis is on obtaining consent as an expression of the patient's autonomy, rather than as a device to avoid being sued, an alternative conceptual model of consent is to view consent as a *threshold* permitting the therapist to treat. Although known risks to treatment would still have to be disclosed, the patient's consent would become a broad agreement to receive therapy which would not require the practitioner to describe the process or consult the patient on each aspect of therapy. This view is essentially contractual, rather than duty-based, and presumes that patients should be free to negotiate on their own terms. This threshold agreement in effect gives patients the autonomy to surrender their autonomy. It impliedly requires the patient to exercise some responsibility for consulting the particular practitioner in the first place. This threshold model should be distinguished from implied consent, which presupposes that the patient, if given all the information, would consent to the procedure in any event. Rather, the threshold model of consent denotes recognition by the patient, as well as the therapist, that aspects of the therapeutic encounter cannot be broken down into neat legalistic categories.

How far this model would work is questionable, particularly in the UK and USA where the law of consent demands that competent patients be appropriately informed of risks and knowingly agree to them. Alternative practitioners should be wary of assuming that there is congruence between themselves and their patients, only to be sued when a predictable risk materialises. What this suggested alternative requires is that the individualised approach to care extends to an individualised approach to information given on the basis of what the particular patient wants. This would allow patients the opportunity to formally waive their autonomy and opt for a beneficence-based model in which the therapist concentrates on healing and the patient concentrates on being healed.

It might seem far-fetched to think that patients would truly wish to deprive themselves of the right to act autonomously when the concept of individualism and individual rights permeates every other aspect of the culture. Nonetheless, the above account may explain why many CAM practitioners do work in an unashamedly paternalistic fashion, which allows the patient a safe, holding space in which mind/body and spirit can be brought back into healthy balance. The notion of autonomy is far from redundant in analysing the CAM relationship, but needs to be reconfigured in a way which reflects the actuality of what CAM therapists do and what CAM patients expect.

Competence requirement

The law of consent is based on the assumption that people have rational decision-making capacity. Although competent adults are, in theory, free to make irrational decisions, the presumption is that, given the appropriate information and absence of coercive influences, rational people will make rational choices. Holistic CAM therapists may, however, have a profoundly different understanding of human functioning which impacts on this element of consent. Fulder argues that the ancient traditions upon which CAM are based transcend the symptom-based, fitness-based, or function-based theories underlying western, reductionist models of health. Rather, the more vitalist and life-orientated themes underpinning alternative therapies give rise to very different ways of describing and indeed conceptualising health:

> ... [H]ealth in Oriental Medicine involves a harmonious relation with all the energies and influences within which man is immersed. These include but are not limited to material, natural, environ-

mental, and social influences. But it also implies having a good constitutional and genetic basis...[3]

Defining health other than by reference to the biomedical paradigm has important consequences for the relatively recent concept of respect for autonomy. As Fulder argues:

> ... [I]t is recognised that health is a mind–body–heart issue, without acknowledging any boundaries between them, Oriental medicine and the major alternative medical systems never passed a Cartesian phase, so there is no need to postulate or evoke concepts like psychosomatic, or even autonomy. These are qualities observed naturally within the mind–body–heart continuum, expressed as the total energetic body of man.[4]

The concepts of rationality and competence depend critically on a dualist understanding of mind and body. They are rooted in present-day culture in which the 'knowing' of the mind is prioritised over the 'knowing' of the body. Yet many CAM practitioners rely on wisdom held in the body to guide their diagnosis and treatment. This, as Cohen argues, has profound implications for legal definitions of competence:

> Applicable legal rules rest on current biomedical and scientific definitions of competency, yet disciplines such as hypnosis and energy healing assert the possibility of communication and consciousness on subtle levels. For instance, through tiny mind–body movements, hypnotherapists can communicate with patients who are in deep trance states or under anaesthesia. The phenomenon of multiple levels of communication in trance states not fully measurable through conventional scientific epistemologies is well known in shamanic traditions.[5]

Using this thesis, it could be argued that CAM therapists cannot and should not separate the patient's conscious will from the rest of their functioning, especially when the therapy may be working at subtle energetic levels which involve different sorts of 'knowing'. Attractive though this line of thinking may be, it would attract little sympathy in a court of law. It may however be a useful basis for explaining to the patient why precise risks cannot be given in the same way as might be expected in a conventional health care relationship. This should not be seen as an excuse not to provide patients with information about risks of treatment *where these are known*. There are many therapeutic disciplines, including those which are based on fundamentally different interpretations of health and disease, in which the risks are known and should be disclosed.

Voluntariness requirement

CAM practitioners can be very persuasive figures and can often assume considerable significance in their patients' lives. Practitioners should avoid overriding the patient's will by imposing their own theories of health and sickness and rejecting the patient's theories as to why they are sick. There is no reason to think that CAM patients are unusually gullible, but practitioners should avoid treatment or lifestyle suggestions which are based wholly on personal opinion and are not supported by evidence. CAM practitioners should respect a patient's right to consult a second opinion and should not try to turn patients against conventional or other medical advice. The notion of voluntariness may be particularly inappropriate where the therapy requires the patient, in a certain sense, to surrender their autonomy. This may be quite explicit, if innocuous, as in the case of a hypnotherapy, or more subtle, as in psychotherapeutic approaches which depend on sacrificing short-term autonomy in the hope of giving the patient longer term freedom to direct their own lives. Concepts of voluntariness as currently understood may need to be thought through where the healing process requires patients to surrender their will to their guru, god or own higher power.

Consent as a product of western, consumerist, individualistic values

A modified version of the above argument provides a further objection to the application of the law of consent to CAM relationships. This objection turns less on the extent to which autonomy of will is a post-Cartesian concept, and more on the extent to which respect for autonomy is an intrinsically western construct which is culture-specific and untranslatable to other contexts. Even in America and Europe, respect for autonomy has only recently been regarded as an essential component of the doctor/patient relationship. Certainly, Hippocratic tradition saw no place for autonomy in the terms we think of it today. As well as its absence from the Hippocratic Oath, the modern idea of autonomy is also absent from early statements of the American Medical Association (AMA) and the World Medical Association (WMA). In his examination of ancient Chinese medical ethics principles, Tsai suggests a reason for this absence:

> Probably this is because patients always come to their doctors for a cure rather than with a conscious concern that their autonomy be respected.[6]

This seemingly obvious point is often overlooked in the autonomy debate. The experience of illness is debilitating and when people are sick their overall autonomy is diminished. This does not mean that patients want major life decisions to be made on their behalf and without consulting them. It may, however, mean that patients assume that they are safe in thinking that qualified health professionals have the knowledge and skills to treat them and that they can trust that the health professional will do whatever is necessary as being in their best interests.

Since a desire to be healed, rather than a desire to be consulted, motivates most patients, should the preoccupation with respect for autonomy be extended to ethical debate outside the American bioethical community, where different cultural norms prevail? Holm argues that American bioethical principles cannot be applied transculturally unless attention is paid to their scope and content:

> Because the theory [of the four principles of medical ethics] is developed from American common morality (and in reality only from a subset of that morality) it will mirror certain aspects of American society, and may, for this reason, be untransferable to other contexts and other societies.[7]

Should autonomy, and by extension consent, be expected to have the same priority in cultures where health care is more beneficence-oriented than autonomy-oriented? A follow-on question, which strikes at the heart of the book, is whether one can expect autonomy and consent to be prioritised in therapies which originate in cultures which do not prioritise the rights of the individual above all else. In essence, can one expect, for example, a Chinese acupuncturist, or a Tibetan healer, or a Japanese shiatsu practitioner to value autonomy if this is anathema to their cultural values?

As a matter of law, practitioners, regardless of their nationality or place of training, will be expected to comply with the laws in which they are practising. Ethically, the question would seem to turn on whether the treatment provided meets the cultural expectations of the client. Patients, it should be remembered, only sue when they receive treatment which falls short of their expectations – including their cultural expectations about the roles of healers and patients. If a practitioner is uncomfortable with giving patients detailed explanations about the therapy, or eliciting the patient's wishes prior to each intervention, then this should be spelt out at the start of the therapeutic encounter, so that individual patients may choose whether they are prepared to enter a therapeutic relationship on this basis.

Notes

1 Holm, S. (1993) 'What Is Wrong With Compliance?' *Journal of Medical Ethics.* 19: 108–110.
2 Vickers, A. and Zollman, C. (1999) 'ABC of Complementary Medicine. Complementary Medicine and the Patient'. *British Medical Journal.* 319: 1486–1489.
3 Fulder, S. (1998) 'The Basic Concepts of Alternative Medicine and Their Impact on Our Views of Health'. *The Journal of Alternative and Complementary Medicine.* 4(2): 147–158.

4   Ibid.
5   Cohen, M. (1998) *Complementary and Alternative Medicine: Legal Boundaries and Regulatory Perspectives.* Johns Hopkins University Press: Baltimore, MD and London.
6   Tsai, D. (1999) 'Ancient Chinese Medical Ethics and the Four Principles of Biomedical Ethics'. *Journal of Medical Ethics.* 25: 315–321.
7   Holm, S. (1995) 'Not Just Autonomy – The Principles of American Biomedical Ethics'. *Journal of Medical Ethics.* 21: 332–338.

13

TRUTH-TELLING

Key ethical issues
- Ethical justifications for truth-telling
- Withholding information in the patient's interests
- Should CAM therapists diagnose patients?

In order to make decisions about their treatment, patients need to know the full picture, and this means being given any information that others have about them. Lying to patients, or deliberately misleading them, prevents them from being able to control their own lives. Health care also involves duties of fidelity and promise-keeping, which involve honest and open communication. A Kantian duty-based theorist would say that it is always necessary to tell the truth, even if this would have disastrous consequences, and that moral agents have an absolute duty to be honest, even if this leads to disastrous consequences. Practitioners, along with the rest of society, tend not to share this categoric point of view.

However, there are also strong consequence-based arguments for telling patients the truth. The health care relationship is predicated on trust. If patients discover, or have reason to think that the person treating them is not telling the truth, this is likely to destroy the trust underpinning the therapeutic relationship. As Holmes and Lindley suggest, telling the truth is even more critical to a relationship in which psychotherapeutic dynamics are operating. They argue:

> Deception jeopardizes the therapeutic process in two ways. First, in the obvious sense that the therapist cannot be sure that she will not be found out, thus destroying the trust a patient must have in her for successful therapy; second, in the sense that deception would undermine the moral authority of a therapist whose work is

predicated on the principle that people should face up to the truth about themselves, even if this is painful.[1]

The virtue of truth-telling, whilst prized in the community at large, is thought to be particularly vital for health professionals who have access to privileged information about the people who consult them. As such, health professionals are in a position of power. There is an implied, if not an express, obligation that health professionals will not abuse that position of power and will not exert control by keeping information from patients which patients have a right to know, or by distorting information to influence decision-making.

Notwithstanding these reasons, the earliest codes of ethics did not include a duty to tell the truth in much the same way that they did not include any explicit requirement to respect patient autonomy. The same social forces that have elevated the principle of respect for autonomy have led to the inclusion of explicit duties of veracity in more recent codes. Yet, considerable ambiguity surrounds how far practitioners should be expected to divulge information to patients. Beauchamp and Childress assert:

> [V]eracity is prima facie binding, not absolute. Non-disclosure, deception and lying will all occasionally be justified when veracity conflicts with other obligations.[2]

In terms of ethical principles, practitioners would be justified in lying or withholding the truth (or the whole truth), when disclosure would conflict with duties of beneficence and non-maleficence. In short, practitioners may judge that it is prudent to be economical with the truth if full disclosure, at that point in time, would do more harm than good. As with other potentially paternalistic actions, the practitioner will only be justified in withholding or distorting information if he or she has a compelling reason for thinking that to do so will, on balance, benefit, rather than harm, the patient.

A chiropractor recommends that a patient with severe back pain asks her doctor to organise an X-ray of her spine. The X-ray reveals that the patient is suffering from a chronic, degenerative bone disease. The chiropractor is quite shocked that the patient does not seem troubled by the diagnosis, especially when the patient tells him that her doctor says that she'll be 'going strong at 90'. The chiropractor is disturbed, as his manual diagnosis of the patient suggests that the disease is at a more advanced stage than the doctor is letting on, and he fears that the effects of this disease will dramatically limit his patient's mobility.

This situation presents a real dilemma for the practitioner. Whilst he does not want to perpetuate the deception, he does not want to make matters worse by contradicting the doctor. In this situation, it is worth recognising that the GP may have a long-standing relationship with the patient, which allows him to be confident that deceiving this particular patient will encourage her to continue to exercise and to keep mobile, which will slow down the progression of the disease. Nonetheless, the chiropractor might feel that the patient would be better served by knowing the full facts, in which case, he would have to weigh up the benefits and disadvantages of full disclosure.

For health professionals, the question of truth-telling usually arises in the context of breaking bad news. The ethical conflict is between the desire to respect people's autonomy and the desire to protect them from harm, specifically, the distress of receiving distressing news. So common is this conflict that a specific term, 'therapeutic privilege', has evolved to describe situations in which a health practitioner decides to withhold information on the basis that it would cause the patient more harm than benefit to be given the information.

Cultural variations

Far from being universal, the desire to acquire knowledge is highly culturally specific. It follows that in the UK and USA, where patient autonomy is highly prized, there might be an expectation and requirement that practitioners tell patients all that they have discovered so that the patient can make choices on the basis of that information. Such a belief relies on a number of assumptions about how people make decisions. In cultures where individual autonomy is paramount, the model is that of the isolated rational being, making logical decisions on the basis of all the information available. In practice, even in societies where autonomy is respected, this does not fully represent how most people make decisions. Most patients are coerced by factors such as the need to return to fitness and thus to work as soon as possible, the views of family and significant others, and a host of irrational or even superstitious beliefs around the meaning of health and illness. In other cultures, the focus is not solely on the individual's autonomy, but also on the role of the immediate family, the extended family and the wider community as decision-makers.

Within mainstream bioethics, paternalism is roundly criticised. However, this view is culturally and contextually specific and may or may not represent the experiences of CAM practitioners and CAM patients. Many cultures feel that patients, who are already depleted by illness, should not be burdened with bad news. Rather, it is felt, they should have their hope bolstered, so that they have a positive mental approach. It is only within the last ten years that this position has begun to change in Japan, where the notion of informed consent was seen to be more harmful to the patient than beneficial. As with respect for autonomy, how far individual patients would want to be told the truth will differ from patient to patient and therapists could usefully discuss this issue with patients prior to history-taking and diagnosis.

Should CAM therapists diagnose?

Although it has been proposed that in order to respect autonomy health professionals should always tell patients the truth, the main situation in which truth-telling becomes an ethical issue is when therapists withhold information about something very serious, such as a diagnosis of terminal cancer. Consider this example given earlier:

> *A reflexologist who suspects that his patient has bowel cancer feels that the patient's spirits are so likely to be damaged by disclosing bad news that he keeps his opinion to himself.*

Here, the therapist is relying on a consequentialist justification to withhold information. His stated reason for not disclosing his fears is that the outcome of this would be to cause undue distress to the patient, although the patient may subsequently feel that it would have been better to have been told, than to have her feelings spared. This outcome-based justification may also be a cover-up for a less acceptable reason. The reflexologist may have decided against sharing his fears because he does not feel that he can cope with the patient's grief, or wants to be spared the trauma of disclosing such bad news. This may highlight a need for therapists to receive better training in communication skills, including how to give patients bad news.

It is also important to ask whether, in the absence of training in conventional medicine, a CAM therapist is even in a position to make such a diagnosis. Many codes of ethics state that CAM practitioners should not diagnose medical conditions. Although, as in the above case, a practitioner may be reasonably confident that a patient is suffering from a particular condition, it would be legitimate to withhold that suspicion, recommending instead that the patient consult his GP or primary health care physician. This is because until the diagnosis has been confirmed, it is arguably not going to benefit a patient to be given bad news which may not even be accurate.

Codes continue to insist that practitioners do not diagnose, but the ambiguity of this requirement is unhelpful, both to practitioners and patients. Manifestly, practitioners who offer to treat physical or psychological symptoms need to be able to make differential diagnoses, either within their own paradigmatic framework or within a conventional understanding. More and more therapists have an extensive training in anatomy and physiology which enables them to diagnose in western terms. Because biomedicine is the dominant cultural paradigm, therapists need to be able to tell patients when they have something wrong with them in a way which is readily understandable.

The language of bad news, of necessity, may need to be the language of the prevailing paradigm. Whether patients would wish to receive that information from the CAM practitioner or a conventional practitioner is again something which practitioners may wish to negotiate with patients before the start of therapy.

Truth-telling and patient-centred practice

In much the same way as consent is viewed in adversarial terms, it might be assumed from the literature that health professionals deliberately withhold information from patients to assert their power or to undermine their autonomy. An alternative way of thinking about truth-telling is to consider the content and pace of information disclosure as more to do with beneficence than autonomy. CAM practitioners may, in certain situations, decide to withhold information or employ deception as a deliberate therapeutic technique. Examples might include homoeopaths who prescribe patients with placebo remedies or psychotherapists who use paradoxical interventions (that is, telling patients the opposite of what they believe to be the case) to provoke them into a new way of thinking about their problems. Such techniques are not necessarily unethical.

Where CAM practitioners are treating holistically, bodies may be amenable to change more readily than minds. In any psychotherapeutic dynamic, the therapist needs to be aware of the point at which the patient is ready to discard previous, unhealthy patterns of behaviour and replace them with healthier models of functioning. The consent model proposed in the previous chapter is consistent with practitioners deciding when and what information should be revealed in the patient's best interests. This presumes an extremely high level of understanding between the practitioner and the patient. The trust involved in the beneficence-based model of patient-centred practice cannot be presumed, but builds up over time. Until that time, practitioner and client may consider explicitly negotiating how information should be disclosed, and at what pace.

Notes

1   Holmes, J. and Lindley, R. (1998) *The Values of Psychotherapy* (revised edition). Karnac Books: London.
2   Beauchamp, T. and Childress, J. (1994) *Principles of Biomedical Ethics* (4th edition). Oxford University Press: New York.

14

CONFIDENTIALITY AND
PATIENT RECORDS

Key ethical issues
* Why respect confidentiality?
* Limits on confidentiality: duty to disclose versus discretion to disclose
* Duty to keep records
* Patients' access to their records
* Data protection requirements

It is often asserted that confidentiality is one of the most important ethical duties of a health care practitioner. Confidentiality is an ethical requirement which is borne out of the patient's expectations of the therapeutic encounter. Patients, it is argued, would not be willing to divulge highly personal information about themselves unless they believed that the practitioner would safeguard that information and use it only for the benefit of that patient. The principle of confidentiality is enshrined in numerous codes and declarations, and is affirmed by the amended Declaration of Geneva (1983), which extends the duty of confidentiality beyond a patient's death. From where does the duty of confidentiality arise and how wide is its scope?

Ethical justifications for respecting confidentiality

The ethical justifications for respecting confidentiality fall into two main categories.[1] The first relies on the concept of confidentiality as being morally valuable in itself, comprising principles such as respect for autonomy and respect for privacy, along with the explicit or implicit promise on the part of the practitioner not to disclose that patient's secrets. The second reason for respecting confidences is based on consequences. A consequentialist would argue that people's health and overall happiness are more likely to be attained if patients are able to make full and frank disclosures to their health carers. Patients are only likely to do this if practitioners do not disclose this information to other people without the patient's permission. Moreover, the consequences of disclosing confidential information will be to destroy the relationship of trust upon which the health care relationship is based.

The following case highlights the dangers of an inadvertent breach of confidentiality:

> *A husband and wife (naturopath and acupuncturist respectively) work at the same natural health clinic. A patient of the wife is very upset when she attends for her weekly appointment because her nephew has been expelled from school for selling drugs. A couple of days later, the husband is treating the sister of his wife's patient, who is mother to the expelled boy. She enters in a highly emotional state and bursts into tears as she takes her coat off. Before she has brought the subject up herself, the husband says how sorry he is to hear about her son and says that this must be a very difficult time for her. His patient is astounded and outraged that he even knows about her problems with her son, especially as she is upset because she has just received a telephone call from a friend who has been diagnosed with cancer. She knows that her sister, to whom she is not particularly close, is a client of her practitioner's wife, and assumes, correctly, that her sister is the source of the information. Both sisters terminate therapy.*

As this case shows, most breaches of confidentiality are not deliberate or intended to cause a patient distress. Often, information is disclosed carelessly, rather than intentionally. This does not make them any less reprehensible.

Practitioners should always protect their patient's confidentiality if they are writing up a case study for publication, or discussing a case at a professional meeting or for teaching purposes. This means withholding the patient's name, and, if necessary, changing irrelevant details to make the patient less identifiable. Therapists who are intending to write about their practice should obtain a prior release for publication from their clients.[2]

Practitioners should make sure that their staff are equally aware of the need to protect patient confidentiality. Since support staff will not be bound by a professional duty of confidentiality, practitioners should ensure that any employees have a confidentiality clause written into their contract of employment.

> *A CAM group practice employs a full-time receptionist. One afternoon, a man telephones to ask whether his wife has arrived for her osteopathic appointment yet, as one of their children is sick and needs to be picked up from school. The receptionist checks the diary and informs the man that his wife has not got an appointment, and adds*

*that she can't recall having seen her for a few months. It subsequently
transpires that the man is not the woman's husband, but a private
investigator, hired by the husband to find out if his wife is having an
affair. The woman makes a complaint to the osteopath's professional
body, who uphold the complaint on the basis that the practitioner is
vicariously liable for the action of his staff.*

As a general rule, CAM practitioners should keep confidential any information they discover about patients or third parties in a professional
capacity. Professional bodies regard confidentiality as a key aspect of good
practice and are likely to punish practitioners severely for breaching confidentiality without good reason. Practitioners should take all necessary steps
to make sure that patient's notes are stored safely and that their staff appreciate that they also owe patients a duty of confidentiality.

Confidentiality: not an absolute duty

Since many patients do not appreciate that the duty of confidentiality is
limited and not absolute, therapists should explicitly tell patients at the
outset of the therapeutic encounter the sorts of situations in which the therapist may have to disclose confidential information about them. There are
some situations where a therapist must divulge information as a matter of
law and other situations where the therapist has the discretion to divulge
information if this is ethically appropriate. A practitioner should be
prepared to justify any disclosure of confidential information. Precise rules
governing confidentiality vary from therapy to therapy and country to
country. All therapists must familiarise themselves with the professional and
legal duties which affect their practice. Practitioners should set out the limits
of confidentiality at the start of the therapeutic encounter so that the
patient can decide whether or not they wish to withhold certain sensitive
information.

When must a therapist divulge information?

Most codes of ethics identify a limited number of situations in which the
therapist must divulge confidential information.

* *In accordance with a statutory provision*: Various statutory provisions
  require information to be divulged. In the UK, this includes statutes
  relating to notifiable disease, notification of drug addiction and notification of venereal diseases (excluding AIDS). Disclosure of notifiable
  diseases should usually be made to the patient's GP (even without their
  consent) who is under a statutory duty to report the information to the
  Community Medical Officer.

- *In accordance with a court order*: A court may subpoena a therapist or a therapist's records if these are thought to be relevant to either civil or criminal proceedings. Therapists are not able to claim that the information was received in professional confidence, but should only disclose the information which is relevant to the proceedings.
- *Where child abuse is suspected*: In the UK, section 47 of the Children Act 1989 requires local authorities to investigate cases where it is suspected that a child in their area is 'suffering or is likely to suffer from serious harm'. Certain agencies, including health authorities, are required to assist 'by providing relevant information and advice'. A CAM therapist who is employed by a health authority may be required to report suspected abuse. A therapist who works in the private sector has a discretion in whether to disclose suspicions, unless her code of ethics requires disclosure of suspected child abuse.

When may a therapist divulge information?

Codes of ethics stipulate other situations in which the therapist may divulge confidential information.

- *Disclosure with the patient's consent*: Since the duty of confidentiality is there to protect the interests and autonomy of the patient, it is legitimate to disclose information with the patient's consent. A patient, for example, who is claiming damages for an industrial injury, may authorise his osteopath to release copies of his clinical records to his employers. In order to prevent a complaint in the future, practitioners might wish to consider seeking written consent from patients before disclosing personal health information about them. Consent should be sought before contacting a client's GP.
- *Disclosure without consent where it is necessary to disclose patient information to other health professionals or in the patient's interests*: Where a practitioner works in a multi-disciplinary setting, it may sometimes be necessary to share information with other health professionals to fulfil their duty of care to the patient.

> *A naturopath is extremely troubled by what appears to be a mass on the patient's tongue. She urges the patient to consult his GP, but the patient refuses. A fortnight later, the mass appears to have grown. The patient still refuses to contact his GP, and will not allow the naturopath to do so.*

The patient is putting the practitioner in a difficult situation by refusing to let her tell the GP. Whilst the practitioner should only go against the patient's wishes in the most extreme circumstances, it may be necessary to decline to treat the patient, especially when the practitioner is sure that the patient has a serious pathology which requires conventional treatment.

- *Where disclosure is necessary to protect the public or a third party from harm*: It will only very rarely be appropriate for a therapist to breach confidentiality in the patient's own interests. A possible situation might be where a practitioner finds out that a patient is intending suicide.

> *A registered herbalist has been treating a twenty-one-year-old manic depressive patient for a year and a half. Although the patient has previously been detained and treated compulsorily, his symptoms are much improved and seem well controlled with herbal treatment. The herbalist has been able to establish a good therapeutic rapport with her client, who clearly trusts her. One week, the patient arrives in tears because he has just been fired from his job. He says that he plans to kill himself. The herbalist does not know whether she should breach the patient's confidentiality and call the police, a social worker or his GP.*

Dimond advises that in such a situation, the practitioner must assess whether the patient is mentally competent. If the patient was not competent, and the practitioner did nothing, she could be failing in her duty of care to the patient. In the above case, the practitioner would have to determine whether the patient was suffering from depression to such a degree that his wishes could be described as non-autonomous. If this were the case, the practitioner should contact the patient's GP. If, however, the practitioner decides that the patient is mentally competent, then the practitioner has no legitimate basis to intervene.[3]

Assessing risk of harm to third parties: what to disclose and when?

Disclosures without consent usually arise when the practitioner is trying to avert harm to a third party. At what point does a therapist decide that a patient constitutes such a threat to a third party that confidentiality ought to be breached? The UK's General Osteopathic Council offer the following advice:

> Disclosures without consent may be necessary in the public interest – when your duty to society overrides your duty to your patients. This will usually happen when such patients put themselves or others at serious risk, for example by the possibility of a violent or criminal act. Even then, you must first make every reasonable effort to persuade the patient to change their behaviour and to disclose

information themselves. If you cannot persuade them to do this you should disclose the information to an appropriate person or authority, taking legal advice first. You must be able, if necessary to justify your actions. [4]

Although this question has not been dealt with by the UK courts, the issue was discussed in the highly influential US *Tarasoff* case.[5]

In 1969, Prosenjit Poddar killed his former girlfriend, Tatiana Tarasoff. Two months earlier, Poddar had confided to his therapist that he wanted to kill Tarasoff when she returned to California after the summer vacation. Poddar was a voluntary out-patient at a hospital forming part of the University of California, Berkeley. At his therapist's request, the police detained Poddar for questioning. The police found him to be rational and released him after he denied he intended to kill Tarasoff and undertook to keep away from her. Poddar did not return to therapy because his therapist had breached his confidentiality. Two months later he went to Tarasoff's home and stabbed and shot her. On appeal, Tarasoff's parents successfully sued the therapist and his supervisor for negligence in failing to warn Tatiana about the danger Poddar posed. The Supreme Court of California upheld their claim, saying that 'protective privilege ends where public privilege begins'.

What was important in this case is that if the therapist had warned Tarasoff or her family, it might have been possible to avert the harm in question. This legal duty to warn third parties of harm severely curtails a therapist's ability to respect their patient's confidentiality. A legal duty to warn is not yet part of UK law, although a practitioner would have discretion to breach confidentiality in such circumstances. There would be less justification to breach the confidentiality of a patient who threatened violence in the abstract. A practitioner needs to feel fairly confident that the threat is genuine and that in breaching confidentiality, preventative action can be taken.

Although AIDS is not a notifiable disease in the UK, similar questions arise in relation to whether a therapist has a right, if not a duty, to disclose a patient's HIV positive status to his or her sexual partner(s). The problem is particularly acute when the sexual partner is also a patient of the therapist, and thus someone to whom the practitioner also owes a duty of care. In this situation, disclosure without the consent of a patient would only be justified where there is a serious and identifiable risk to a specific individual who, if not so informed, would be exposed to infection.

A homoeopath has treated a husband and wife separately for several years. The husband, who, unbeknownst to his wife, is bisexual, has just found out that he is HIV positive, and has come to the homoeopath for support. The homoeopath encourages him to tell his wife about his status, but he refuses to do so. The homoeopath is aware that his wife is trying to get pregnant. After repeated attempts to encourage his patient to tell her, the homoeopath takes the matter into her own hands and informs the wife. The wife tests negative for HIV, but leaves her husband.

Undoubtedly, such a disclosure would constitute a breach of confidentiality, but in all probability a disciplinary body or court would hold such a breach was justified in the public interest. In cases such as these, the practitioner must decide whether their duty lies in respecting a client's confidences or protecting others from harm. The practitioner must also weigh up the consequences of her actions. Ideally, a disclosure should bring about more good than harm, although it may not be possible to predict the eventual outcome.

Most practitioners recognise the centrality of respecting patients' confidences and a decision to breach confidentiality may cause the practitioner anxiety and concern. Disclosure is only justified if it will achieve the greater good of protecting the public. There are two main points if a therapist feels that disclosure is unavoidable. The first is that the therapist must tell the patient that he or she intends to make the disclosure and to tell the patient to whom the disclosure will be made. Wherever possible, practitioners should seek the patient's consent to the disclosure. The second requirement is that the disclosure should be able to achieve its purpose and should be limited to the minimum disclosure consistent with this.

In a UK case, doctors wished to divulge the contents of a psychiatric report which had been commissioned by a detained psychiatric patient, W, with a view to securing his release. W was detained in a secure hospital without time limit after killing five people and seriously injuring two more. In the event, far from recommending his early release, the report by Dr Egdell suggested that the detainee was even more dangerous than first thought. The patient sought to block its disclosure, arguing that since he had commissioned the report, he should be able to suppress it. Dr Egdell, who felt that the contents of the report should be made known to the relevant authorities, sent a copy to the hospital director and to the Home Office. W brought an action against Dr Egdell for breach of confidence. When the case went to trial, it was agreed that it was right and proper to make such disclosure against the patient's wishes.[6]

The court nonetheless made it clear that the balance of public interest clearly lay in the restricted disclosure of vital information to the relevant authorities, but that this would not have justified the doctor in that case disclosing his report, say, to a newspaper.

Disclosure of confidential information is particularly troublesome within psychotherapy, where the therapist may have doubts about the veracity of the patient's account, and where patient notes are likely to include the therapist's interpretations. The American Psychiatric Association's 1985 Code provides guidance which may be useful for other therapists:

> Ethically, the psychiatrist may disclose only that information which is relevant to a given situation. He/she should avoid offering speculation as fact. Sensitive material such as an individual's sexual orientation or fantasy material is usually unnecessary.[7]

Record-keeping

In order to benefit patients, therapists need to have a clear record of the patient's history and previous treatment. Therapists should keep accurate records of all consultations with clients. Details of any advice given over the telephone should also be recorded accurately and contemporaneously. Legally, if a therapist is challenged in court, records will serve as vital evidence as to what course of action the therapist took, and why. As well as having legal ramifications, there are strong ethical reasons for why accurate, contemporaneous records should be taken. Primarily, written records serve as an integral part of the professional decision-making process. Although a therapist may make a tentative diagnosis, it is vital to keep accurate records from each session so that the therapist can review how the patient's symptom profile is changing, and whether an initial diagnosis may need to be modified in the light of further evidence. Records should contain the following information:

- the date of the visit;
- the patient's account of how they have been since the last visit;
- the therapist's observations based on what the client has said, physical observations, etc.;
- any additional comments by the patient, including disagreement with the practitioner's views;
- the course of action pursued by the therapist in terms of treatment given, remedy prescribed, etc.;
- any recommendations made to the patient in terms of diet, exercise, etc.;
- any recommendation that the patient contact his or her GP/primary health physician.

Therapists should remember that records may be inspected by other people at some time in the future. They may even be used as evidence in court. They should never include disparaging remarks, or comments which are liable to misinterpretation at a later date. In the case of handwritten notes, if a correction is necessary, the original should be crossed out, and the amendment made alongside it with the therapist's initials and the date. This will look a lot less suspicious than using correcting fluid. Computer notes should also not be altered retrospectively.

Should therapists allow patients to see their own records?

Many therapists would be nervous of allowing patients access to their notes, and would draw on the medical model in which patients are not generally encouraged to do this and may only access them in accordance with the formal procedure laid down by statute. Therapists might ask themselves whether this is for any genuine therapeutic reason, or is merely a vestige of medical paternalism; that notes belong to the practitioner and the patient doesn't need to see them. Therapists are most likely to be concerned when the notes include, in addition to what the patient has actually said, the therapist's observations, not all of which may be flattering to the patient, particularly when talking about the patient's mental state. Here, it is critical that the therapist distinguishes between what the patient has said and what is conjecture. Specifically, if the therapist is interpreting the information given by the patient, it would be wise to record this in such a way that it is obvious that this is a working hypothesis.

From a patient's point of view, since the records contain information about them, they may feel very strongly that they should be allowed to access these records. They may legitimately feel that they own their records. Patients may wish to see their notes to make sure that the therapist has written down what they have said in a way which captures the essence of what they were trying to get across. Indeed, to the extent that CAM therapists should be encouraging and promoting self-responsibility, there may be very strong reasons for making patients responsible for their own notes. Featherstone and Forsyth describe how such a model might work in practice:

> Every person holds their own health book. It contains all the infor-
> mation regarding their medical history, treatments received, health
> assessments and expert reports. During any contact with a health
> professional, notes will be entered into the book, as well as exami-
> nation results. At any time, the person may add comments and
> observations, which may include disagreement with the expert's
> picture. Their health records are their personal property and
> responsibility.[8]

Featherstone, a CAM practitioner who attempted to introduce this model into her own practice, found that patient record-holding was not without its problems, and that many patients would forget to bring their health book to their consultation. Confusion could also arise if the patient were consulting different therapists concurrently, several of whom may be treating within different – and potentially irreconcilable – diagnostic frameworks. Practitioners might also have reservations about moving to such a system. A legitimate concern is that since patient records may be used as legal documents in the event of litigation, the practitioner should retain a copy for the length of time within which a complaint can be made in law.

Additionally, records provide the practitioner with a comprehensive, written reminder of the patient's condition and what treatment has been given, so that if patients did forget to bring their notes with them, they might not be able to provide appropriate follow-up treatment. For these reasons, even if practitioners were prepared to let patients keep a duplicate set of their notes, they would probably be advised to keep the original set themselves. Nonetheless, the model is a useful reminder that however patient-centred CAM practitioners like to think they are, they may still be a long way from a genuine model of patient self-responsibility.

Data protection requirements

All records containing personal information about patients need to be kept confidential. Practitioners need to be familiar with the data protection legislation in their own country. In the UK, the law governing data protection has been extended to cover both manually written and computerised records.[9] The relevant legislation is the Data Protection Act 1998. The Act includes osteopaths, chiropractors, and art and music therapists employed by a health authority as 'health professionals' for the purposes of the Act, meaning that these therapists must register with the Office of Data Protection as 'data users'. The Act sets out eight principles. It requires:

- that data be collected and processed fairly and lawfully;
- that data should be held only for specified, lawful registered purposes;
- that data should be used only for registered purposes or disclosed to registered recipients;
- that data should be adequate and relevant to the purpose for which they are held;
- that data should be accurate and, where necessary, kept up to date;
- that data should be held no longer than is necessary for the stated purpose;
- that data should be stored with appropriate security;
- that data subjects should have a right of access to records held on them.[10]

The purpose of the data protection principles is to ensure that patients know what data are held about them, are able to access those data, and are able to correct any inaccuracies. Other CAM professionals should incorporate data protection principles into their practice even though they do not yet fall within the statutory definition of a 'health professional'. If practitioners disclose confidential patient information in breach of the Act, they may have their registration as a 'data user' removed and may no longer have the right to retain information about their patients.

Data should only be used for the purposes for which they were originally collected. In the case of patient records, this primarily means for the purpose of treating the patient. This prohibits a therapist from using sensitive patient information for personal gain, for example, selling information about patients' treatment to a herbal manufacturer.

Under the Act, access to health records may be refused where the health professional responsible for the patient's clinical care thinks that access to the data would be likely to cause serious harm to the physical or mental health of the data subject, or where access would breach the confidences of third parties. Where, rarely, the practitioner genuinely believes it would do more good than harm for the patient to access their notes, a detailed explanation should be given rather than a blanket refusal. CAM practitioners should allow patients access to their notes without a reason, and without charge (other than covering the cost of copying the notes).

Notes

1 For detailed discussion, see Beauchamp, T.L. and Childress, J.F. (1994) *Principles of Biomedical Ethics* (4th edition). Oxford University Press: New York.
2 Jenkins, P. (1997) *Counselling, Psychotherapy and the Law*. Sage: Thousand Oaks, CA, London and New Delhi.
3 Dimond, B. (1998) *The Legal Aspects of Complementary Therapy Practice*. Churchill Livingstone: Edinburgh.
4 General Osteopathic Council (1988) *Pursuing Excellence. Good Practice for Osteopaths*. General Osteopathic Council: London.
5 *Tarasoff* v *Regents of the University of California* 529 P 2d 55 (Cal,1974).
6 *W* v *Egdell* [1990] 1 All ER 107.
7 Cited in Holmes, J. and Lindley, R. (1998) *The Values of Psychotherapy* (revised edition). Karnac Books: London.
8 Featherstone, C. and Forsyth, L. (1997) *Medical Marriage: The New Partnership Between Orthodox and Complementary Medicine*. Findhorn Press: Findhorn, Scotland.
9 The Data Protection Act 1998 ratifies the Council of Europe's *Convention for the Protection of Individuals with regard to Automatic Processing of Personal Data*. This facilitates a common standard of protection for individuals to enable the free flow of information across international boundaries.
10 See Dimond, op. cit.

15

NEGOTIATING CONTRACTS WITH PATIENTS

Key ethical issues
- Achieving security whilst avoiding legalistic relationships
- Rights and responsibilities of both parties
- Role in establishing boundaries
- Terminating therapeutic relationships

Most CAM therapeutic relationships operate within the private sector. Unlike state-provided health care systems, where treatment is either provided free at the point of delivery or via health insurance, most CAM patients have a direct contractual relationship with their therapist, who agrees to provide care usually in return for fees. The force of a contract is that it is a legally binding agreement and either side can sue the other party for being in breach of the contract terms. The reality is that very few patients are dissatisfied to the point of suing their practitioner. Nonetheless, contracts are a vital tool for ensuring that both practitioner and patient know what they are bargaining for.[1] Within the traditional health care setting, contracting with clients has been mostly used in the mental health and psychotherapy field as a way of increasing patient participation and maximising their autonomy. CAM practitioners committed to patient-centred practice might reflect on the value of contracting with patients.

A vital, if uncomfortable, aspect of negotiating the contract is ensuring that the practitioner and patient are sufficiently well suited to pursue a therapeutic relationship. This can only be achieved through good communication at the outset of therapy. In order that the patient knows what they are getting into, practitioners must be explicit about how they work, the scope and style of their practice and the principles which inform their therapeutic bias. Both sides of the contract should be clear about what the therapy can and cannot deliver. Practitioners, whilst being sensitive to individual client needs, should not allow themselves to be manipulated, as in the following case study.

*A recently qualified hypnotherapist is attempting to build up his prac-
tice. A new client wants help to give up smoking. In negotiating how
many sessions may be necessary, the client says that he wants to come
as often as possible, so that rapid progress can be made. The practitioner reckons that the client's need for control and impatience is part
of his pathology, and usually sees clients no more than once a week.
The client is quite insistent that he wishes to come three times a week.
The hypnotherapist eventually agrees to go along with this, partly
because he does not think that the extra sessions will actively harm
the client, but also, in part, because he does not want to lose a potential client and could use the extra income.*

Although this point is acknowledged, no-one has really considered what
each party should do if they feel that they are unable to work with the other.
The first concern is the unhappy patient. What should a patient do if he is
attending for the first time, and takes an instant dislike to the therapist and
decides that he really is not comfortable, and does not even wish to be physically examined by this therapist? However much one says that patients are
entitled to reject a therapist they are not comfortable with, it would take a
brave person to terminate the relationship before it has even commenced,
and furthermore, to refuse to pay for an initial session. Most clients would
simply put up with an initial consultation, pay their money, and simply
never come back again. To avoid this situation, therapists should consider
offering a pre-consultation, so that the patient has an opportunity to find
out a bit about the therapist and meet them before having to commit to
entering therapy. Thought needs to be given as to who should bear the cost
of this meeting. If this is not possible, practitioners should at least be
prepared to spend some time on the telephone with a prospective client, so
that the patient can glean sufficient information to decide whether they want
to enter into a therapeutic relationship.

What of the therapist who feels unable to work with the particular
patient? Therapists have a duty to treat all actual and prospective clients
fairly and in a non-discriminatory fashion, but this does not imply that practitioners have a duty to take on clients with whom they do not feel they will
be able to have a constructive therapeutic relationship. This situation will
arise from time to time and it is important to recognise that it is not just the
patient's autonomy which is important, but the therapist's as well, and there
is no reason for a therapist to be expected to put up with a situation which is
compromising his or her autonomy or integrity.

In most circumstances, a therapist who feels that further work with a
particular patient is impossible and wishes to end the therapeutic relationship prematurely should attempt to explain why he or she is doing this, and
to provide the patient with the name and contact point for an alternative
therapist, or choice of alternatives. The only circumstance in which a thera-

pist should not feel obligated to do this is if the patient's behaviour poses such an immediate and direct threat or assault to the therapist's well-being, for example, the patient physically attacks the therapist, the therapist's sense of personal safety is compromised and the patient's behaviour has effectively unilaterally ended the relationship. In such a situation, the practitioner should make an accurate note of why the relationship ended and any steps taken to minimise an adverse impact on the patient.

Avoiding legalistic relationships with patients

A key element of the therapeutic relationship is the patient's agreement to treatment. It has been argued previously, that there are difficulties in applying legalistic notions of informed consent to relationships between CAM practitioners and their clients. Cohen argues that consent is a poor substitute for well-formed agreements between parties:

> [S]tructuring relationships between provider and patient to clarify roles and expectations about healing methods and outcomes provides a clearer, contractual means by which parties can expand treatment choices to include complementary and alternative medicine. Such an approach encourages the use of holistic modalities in a non-reductionist manner, i.e. to nourish, stimulate and balance vital energy, rather than to treat biomedically defined pathology.[2]

Mutual rights and responsibilities

It has been suggested that CAM therapeutic encounters differ from conventional health care relationships to the extent that CAM practitioners expect patients to exercise self-responsibility. Certainly, the threshold model of consent proposed earlier requires patients to demonstrate a high level of discernment in their initial choice of therapist. Although lip service is paid to the notion of patient self-responsibility, what might be the mutual obligations arising in a contractually based therapeutic encounter?

Patient's responsibilities

- To attend appointments.
- To consider reasonable advice given by the therapist, for example, as to exercise and changes in lifestyle, and to introduce such changes as are possible.
- To pay for missed sessions, if this has been agreed at the outset of therapy.

185

- To respect the therapist's personal and professional boundaries and rights as an individual.

Therapist's responsibilities

- To agree a fee per session (the first session may be more expensive, as this initial appointment may be considerably longer than future appointments), and to set out whether fees will have to be paid for non-attendance.
- To discuss how many sessions before progress is reviewed.
- To indicate the time scale therapy is likely to require before assessing whether there has been any benefit.
- To state the patient's right to terminate the therapeutic relationship at any time.
- To indicate whether the therapist provides any back-up service in case the patient needs to make contact between appointments.
- To discuss any provisions the therapist will make in the sense of providing locum cover during sickness/holidays and to let the patient know in advance if any major interruption to therapy is imminent (for example, extended holiday or maternity leave).
- To supply the patient with a copy of notes or a resumé of treatment, given at the end of therapy, so that patient can use this in the future, when pursuing other/further therapy.
- To disclose whether the practitioner has a supervisor with whom confidential information will be discussed and details of any other situations in which the patient's confidentiality may be breached.

Written versus oral contracts

In most business settings, a contract is a written agreement. This is because both parties to the agreement need to have an accurate record of what the mutual responsibilities are under the contract, and what provisions are in place should either party default. Such legalistic terminology is generally inappropriate in CAM negotiations. Usually, it will be fairly obvious to each party that the client agrees to pay the therapist an agreed sum in return for therapeutic services. Other arrangements may also give rise to a legally binding agreement, for example, practitioners who swap agree to swap treatments with each other, without money changing hands. Practitioners should make it clear when they are treating friends and neighbours whether they are giving treatment as a gift, for which there would be no recompense if the practitioner accidentally caused harm, or as a professional encounter, giving rise to legal responsibilities.

An aromatherapist offers to give her neighbour a massage, because the neighbour had kindly sewn some curtains for her. This is a one-off session, intended as a gift.

An osteopath agrees, in advance, to give his neighbour six osteopathic sessions in return for his neighbour agreeing to landscape his garden. Unfortunately, during the course of one session, the osteopath causes his neighbour a stress fracture. The neighbour successfully sues the osteopath.

What is important in a contractual situation is that each party intends to create legal relations. This means that either side can enforce their obligations, if necessary, in a court of law. For this reason, practitioners and patients may feel that there is value in setting out the terms of engagement. One copy of this document can be given to the patient to take away and keep and another copy can be retained by the therapist along with the patient's notes.

Express terms versus implied terms

A written contract will include specific obligations on the part of the therapist and the client. These are known as express terms. Other aspects of the agreement are sometimes left out, usually because they are so obvious that they do not need to be stated (for example; 'The practitioner hereby agrees not to verbally, physically or emotionally abuse the client...'). Occasionally, a dispute may arise where the parties have not made an express provision. In such a situation, the common law may imply a term into the contract if this is necessary to make sense out of it. In deciding whether an implied term is appropriate, the court would ask whether a hypothetical 'officious bystander', if faced with the disagreement, would automatically write such a clause into the contract.

A student pays an agreed sum of money to be allowed to attend as many yoga classes as she likes for a three-month period. Ten weeks into the three months, she is sent abroad on business for three months. When she returns, she insists that the studio allow her to use up her final two weeks worth of classes. The studio say that this is unreasonable, since the student had 'got her money's worth' out of the studio during the ten weeks and that they cannot be expected to allow students extra classes just because they are away on business any more than they would if a student were ill.

In such a disagreement, the test would be whether an officious bystander would say: 'Of course the agreement implies that missed sessions can be made up', or, as is more likely, 'Of course the student can't make up the missed time'. Practitioners should try to pre-empt this sort of situation by making full provision for payment and absences in the contract.

Privity of contract

Once parties have agreed to enter into a contractual relationship, the doctrine of privity of contract arises. This means that only the parties to the agreement can sue under the contract. Accordingly, if a patient fails to pay her fees, the practitioner cannot sue the patient's husband, since he is not a party to the contract. By a similar token, if a patient has paid in advance for six massage sessions, but decides after one session that she does not like the masseur, she cannot insist that her husband be allowed to use up the remaining sessions. If a therapeutic relationship causes harm, in contract law, only the patient can bring a legal action. In rare situations, a third party may witness the practitioner causing the patient harm. Very occasionally, bystanders may be able to sue someone for negligence in causing them nervous shock.

A woman takes her frail, eighty-year-old mother to a chiropractor. At her mother's request, the woman comes in to the treatment room. She is horrified when the chiropractor twists her mother's head so violently that she causes her to suffer a stroke. Both mother and daughter successfully sue the practitioner.

Terminating the therapeutic relationship

From an ethical point of view, the principles of beneficence and non-maleficence require termination of the therapeutic relationship to be handled with sensitivity. Various questions arise, which practitioners might like to reflect upon:

- Whose decision should it be when to end therapy – the therapist's, the client's or a joint decision?
- In the absence of clearly defined end-points, who decides whether the therapy has been successful (or unsuccessful)?
- Is there any scope for continuing the therapeutic relationship at the patient's request even if the practitioner feels that s/he has done all that is possible for the client?

In the event of a practitioner having to terminate all therapeutic relationships due to unforeseen circumstances, arrangements should be made to ensure that there is continuity of care for a client. Traynor and Clarkson advise:

In the event of the psychotherapist's unplanned termination of contract there is a caretaking responsibility. Clients are precious human beings who entrust themselves to our care and may be in various stages of vulnerability. They confide in us, and their records and psychological processes should be safeguarded. It is appropriate professional practice to take responsibility for the client in these circumstances, and to ensure that arrangements are made that are mindful of their continuing psychological journey and which protect confidentiality.[3]

All practitioners should remember that their duty of confidentiality persists even after the therapeutic relationship has ended. Traynor and Clarkson advise that when a client leaves practice, therapists should go through their notes, removing the client's name and other identifying material. The notes can be given a number and cross indexed, so that they can be relocated if the patient returns to therapy, Therapists should also make arrangements for what will happen to their patients in the event of their death, ideally arranging for a trusted therapist colleague to be an executor for matters relating to one's professional practice.

Notes

1   For further discussion, see Thistle, R. (1998) *Counselling and Psychotherapy in Private Practice*. Sage: Thousand Oaks, CA, London and New Delhi.
2   Cohen, M. (1998) *Complementary and Alternative Medicine: Legal Boundaries and Regulatory Perspectives*. Johns Hopkins University Press, Baltimore, MD and London.
3   Traynor, B. and Clarkson, P. (2000) 'What Happens if a Psychotherapist Dies?' In Clarkson, P. *Ethics. Working with Ethical and Moral Dilemmas in Psychotherapy*. Whurr Publishers: London.

16

DUTIES TOWARDS CHILDREN AND MENTALLY INCAPACITATED ADULTS

Key ethical issues
- Proxy decision-making and the scope of 'best interests'
- Complementary or alternative approaches for seriously ill children
- Children as autonomous decision-makers
- Duties towards mentally incapacitated adults

Amid concerns over the safety of vaccinations and ill-effects of antibiotics, many parents are critical of orthodox medicine and are becoming more open to using complementary approaches for their children. Reasons for this may include the perception that CAM is generally safer and has fewer side effects than orthodox medicine. CAM therapies are perceived as being particularly helpful in treating children suffering from chronic and environmentally-induced conditions, such as asthma, eczema and allergies. Parents of children using CAM for these conditions have often exhausted conventional routes before turning to CAM as a last resort.

There are no precise data on the proportion of CAM practitioners treating children or the range of conditions they treat. It can be assumed, however, that as the percentage of any population using CAM therapies increases, at least a proportion of that usage is going to represent the treatment of children under 16. Most codes of ethics include a provision that children under 16 should not be seen unless a parent or guardian is present, although little rationale is given for this. Therapists need to be aware of the ethical issues raised by treating children. These include: working with parents as proxy decision-makers for non-autonomous children; working with children who are able to make their own decisions; issues of confidentiality relating to children; and risk/benefit ratios involved in using untested remedies on children.

Proxy decision-making

Most health care decisions concerning young children are made by their parents who act as proxy decision-makers. The reasoning behind this is that young children are not thought to be sufficiently autonomous to make their own decisions and so depend upon others to make important decisions for them. In all decisions relating to children, the welfare of the child is of paramount concern. The role of parents is to make good decisions for their children to enable them to reach a stage of maturity when they will be able to decide for themselves. Parents are vested with proxy decision-making powers because it is assumed that they have their child's best interests at heart. Parents (or those vested with parental responsibility) are empowered to take a whole range of health decisions relating to their child's health, from ordinary, everyday issues, such as diet and vaccinations, through to the most grave decisions, such as whether to pursue active therapy in the event of requiring a transplant or cancer therapy.

In order to make health care decisions about their children, parents have to be given adequate information so that they can validly consent. As with adults consenting on their own behalf, parents must be competent to make the decision, and they should not be coerced. As well as consenting to treatment, parents can (in theory, at least) refuse consent to treatment, although in practice, parents tend to be heavily influenced by the advice of the experts caring for their child.

Acting in children's best interests

In most common law jurisdictions, the parental right to consent to or refuse treatment is subject to the *'best interests'* principle. This means that parents have to make decisions which will not only benefit their children, but will be in their child's best interests. It is far from clear what it means to act in a child's best interests. Although this is commonly taken to mean their best *medical* interests, many of the decisions taken by parents are justified on the basis of a combination of *medical and social* interests, or on the basis of the medical and social interests *of the family unit as a whole*. It is this extended understanding of best interests which has justified, for example, parents being allowed to consent to the use of the organs from one child being donated to an ill sibling. Although this could not be said to be in the former child's best medical interests, one can see how social and familial interests are served by not allowing another sibling to die.

One can think of various situations in which children are subjected to interventions which, if not in their best medical interests, are thought not to be against their interests. Male circumcision is an example of an intervention which may not be in the child's best medical interests but is regarded by some as acceptable as being in the child's best social interests if the family consider circumcision important to their religious or cultural traditions.

Allowing children to participate in minimally invasive research trials (such as unobtrusive observation or anonymous epidemiological research) is another example of a situation which will not benefit the child directly, but is thought to be of social value, so long as it is not going to harm the child. Consideration of these examples are central to our analysis, since it may be possible to argue that use of alternative therapies for children can be construed as being legally and ethically acceptable if it tallies with the parents' value system.

Choosing CAM for children

What is far from clear is the extent to which parents can choose alternative therapies for their children, particularly if this child is seriously ill and there is little evidence to substantiate the use of the therapeutic intervention proposed. Why this is important is because the right to make parental decisions may be removed from parents if they are thought to be acting in a manner that might seriously harm their child. As Barton and Douglas point out:

> The state's interest in the protection of its more vulnerable citizens may require compulsory intervention in the family. Where different lifestyles and modes of child upbringing can no longer be regarded as legitimate within a range of acceptable practices, the family may become an object of scrutiny and judgment as well as assistance.[1]

Liberal democracies recognise that there is considerable diversity in how parents choose to bring up their children and tend to respect that diversity provided it is not inconsistent with respecting the child's welfare. Cultural and religious diversity are taken into account and it is not the role of the state to supplant parental choice in this matter. Describing this issue of choice as a 'fundamental liberty interest', Neeley, commenting on the position in the USA, observes that:

> Accordingly, the parent is also generally free to pursue spiritual means of healing alone for her child and may thus eschew more 'conventional' forms of health care. In fact, a majority of states provide exemptions to their child abuse and neglect laws for spiritual treatment.[2]

He describes how Christian Scientists claim to have evidence of healing which is 'real, frequent and often not explainable under ordinary medical rubrics', but juxtaposes this with studies of increased mortality amongst Christian Scientist schools and colleges.[3] He goes on to raise arguably the most contentious point in this entire issue, namely, that if spiritual healing is not based upon a scientific paradigm, 'there may be no conceptually adequate and unbiased means of comparing methodologies'. Sadly, Neeley is unable to offer any solution to what he describes as the 'paradigmatic acrimony between science and religious faith'. This is regrettable, because the right to choose CAM for children raises fundamental questions about individual rights and freedoms versus collective rights and freedoms, and who should be designated as ultimate decision-maker. This is a critical question for CAM, because the freedom to pursue religious and cultural diversity does not readily extend to the freedom of parents to pursue alternative worldviews if this challenges prevailing orthodoxies.

Any course of action which jeopardises a child's well-being may become a matter for the court. This includes situations in which parents' cultural or religious beliefs put their child's health at risk. Courts are understandably conservative where the life of a child is at stake. Although a large degree of religious freedom is tolerated, courts have been willing to override parental wishes and sanction blood transfusions for children of Jehovah's Witnesses.[4]

What has been the subject of less discussion is how far parental preference for alternative medicine is consistent with a child's best interests. In ethical terms, this raises profound issues about parental autonomy and freedom to raise children in a way which is congruent with their own values. This, in turn, raises questions of whether parental autonomy is something which should be treated potentially as being at odds with the child's interests, or, as Bridgeman argues, something which is more likely to be motivated by:

> considerations of care, obligation and appreciation of interdependence, rather than the application of abstract concepts of conflicting and competing rights.[5]

Children as autonomous decision-makers

Many practitioners are unaware of the precise point at which a child can be treated as sufficiently mature to receive treatment without their parent being present. The prohibition contained in codes of ethics not to treat children under 16 is unnecessarily cautious, as many children under 16 will be competent to consent to CAM treatment. In English law, children over that age are able to make their own medical decisions. The Family Law Reform Act 1969 states at section 8(1):

> The consent of a minor who has attained the age of 16 to any surgical, medical or dental treatment which, in the absence of consent, would constitute a trespass to his person, shall be as effective as it would be if he were of full age; and where a minor has by

virtue of this section given an effective consent to any treatment it shall not be necessary to obtain any consent for it from his parent or guardian.

There is no reason to think that this act does not extend to CAM treatment. The same Act goes on to preserve any common law right that might have existed prior to its passing for children under 16 to consent to treatment. In the UK, the position relating to treatment of minors changed dramatically after the *Gillick* case in 1985. This landmark House of Lords' decision held that the parental right to make decisions for their children, including decisions about medical treatment, yields to the child's right to make his or her own decisions as and when they have sufficient maturity and intelligence to understand fully what is proposed.

This approach, subsequently affirmed by the Children Act 1989 and the UN Declaration of Children's Rights, recognises that competence to make health care decisions is not a matter of status which a child acquires on his or her sixteenth birthday, but depends on the understanding of the individual of the specific decision which needs taking. Although subsequent legal rulings have retreated from the rights of children to refuse as well as consent to treatment, ethically, it is clear that children under 16 may demonstrate sufficient competence to make their own decisions.

In the UK at least then, there may be situations where a CAM practitioner feels that the child is capable of fully understanding the risks which are involved and the nature and purpose of the proposed treatment and is therefore able to give consent in their own right. Because the decision-making ability depends on the nature of the question being asked, it follows that children under 16 are more likely to be able to give their consent to relatively minor interventions than to treatment for acute conditions. The age at which children can be regarded as sufficiently mature enough to make decisions independently is a matter to be assessed by the individual therapist. Current research suggests that children can consent to even quite serious interventions from a surprisingly early age.

Occasionally, a practitioner may be put into conflict with his or her regulatory body if there is a blanket prohibition against treating under 16s on their own, yet the practitioner feels that a child is competent to make her own decisions.

A fifteen-and-a-half-year-old girl consults a homoeopath wishing to receive treatment for a yeast infection. The homoeopath takes a history and establishes that the girl is sexually active and has most probably been infected by her boyfriend. The homoeopath is faced with a dilemma, as the girl is under the age of consent, and the homoeopath does not wish to condone under-age sex. At the same time, she does not want to refuse the girl treatment. In the end, she persuades the girl to return the next day with her partner, who also needs treatment to prevent cross-infection.

In such a case, the practitioner will have to decide what is the most ethical course of action in all of the circumstances. In this particular face, she feels that the girl fully understands the nature and side effects of the treatment, and decides that the girl's willingness to return with her boyfriend suggests sufficient maturity for the homoeopath to be able to regard her as sufficiently autonomous to treat.

Practically, there are probably few situations in which therapists would be likely to see children without their parents since very few children would be likely to be able to afford to consult a therapist on their own, given that most therapeutic encounters operate within the private sector.

Another justification for imposing an age limit of 16 is that some CAM practitioners place considerable emphasis on the patient's need to exercise self-responsibility. Many therapists insist that optimal therapeutic outcomes require the active engagement and participation of their patients. In reality, this usually amounts to advice on lifestyle issues, such as diet and exercise. Whilst children under 16 may be emotionally mature and able to understand what is required of them, they may lack the financial independence to effect these changes. Nonetheless, practitioners may consider that in the particular circumstances, a young person is entitled to privacy and confidentiality and that successful treatment requires parents not to be present. In such situations, the practitioner must document these reasons and be prepared to justify them in the event of disciplinary proceedings.

Benefiting and not harming: children and CAM research

Medical treatment for children is generally under-researched. This is recognised to be a problem in relation to conventional medical treatment, where many drugs are not tested in children. Many of the treatments prescribed for children have not been specifically licensed for such use.[6] Part of the reason for this is that research, by its very nature, cannot be described as being in a patient's best interests. Even if the therapy is subsequently proven to be beneficial, the whole point of research is to test that hypothesis. Applying the 'best interests' test, this means that, strictly speaking, parents cannot consent to their child's participation in even a therapeutic trial (that is, one which is intended to benefit the participants) because, at the time of enrolment, it is not known whether the treatment will prove to be in their best interests. Similarly, research ethics committees (IRBs), which are charged with the duty of protecting research subjects, should not approve research trials on children if the research could be carried out on adults.

This presents something of a paradox. Unless it is permissible to conduct research in children, treatments cannot be designed which will be of specific benefit to them. Children do not necessarily absorb and metabolise therapeutic products in the same way as adults, so it is not appropriate simply to provide children with adult drugs with the dosage reduced proportionate to body mass. Also, there are certain childhood diseases which do not occur in adults, where the research could only be carried out on children suffering from the condition in question. Accordingly, relevant professional codes tend to permit therapeutic research in children provided the research is thought to constitute no more than minimal risk of harm.

Although there is some research into use of CAM in children, particularly for treatment of asthma and skin conditions, generally this area is extremely under-researched. Ethically, this is highly problematic, since in the absence of systematically collected evidence, it may be hard to state with any certainty that a CAM intervention will benefit and not harm a child. Whilst the same is true for adults, this is less problematic because it is generally thought that competent, autonomous adults are entitled to take risks with their own health and are free to make ill-informed or even irrational choices.[7] For children, however, parents have to make decisions which are in their best interests, or, at the very least, which do not expose them to anything greater than minimal harm.

There remains a strong, if unspoken, assumption that where the condition is more critical, patients should at least seek a conventional medical diagnosis before embarking on CAM treatment. Nowhere are these arguments more acute than in relation to the use of CAM for children with serious medical conditions. Whereas adults are free to experiment with their own health, the consensus is that, where orthodox treatment exists, children should be given the best conventional care available. Thus, GPs and the media might support the use of homoeopathy for treating a child's earache, but would almost certainly condemn the use of faith healing as the sole treatment against a child's leukaemia. Whilst CAM therapies may generally be safe and have few side effects, the lack of research threatens the legitimacy of choosing CAM for children.

Mentally incapacitated adults

The duty to respect autonomy presupposes that the patient is an autonomous, competent adult. In the case of mentally incapacitated adults, as with children, practitioners have a duty to act in that person's best interests. Whereas parents are empowered to consent or refuse treatment on behalf of their incompetent children, practitioners themselves have to decide whether their treatment is in the best interests of a mentally incompetent adult.

CAM practitioners may treat mentally incapacitated patients in a variety of contexts. They may be asked to treat adults with learning disabilities, unconscious patients, people who have suffered a stroke, patients suffering from severe depression or other mental disorders or patients suffering from dementia. Often, the request to see such patients will come from the patient's carer or legal guardian. The principle of respect for autonomy requires therapists to respect whatever decision-making capacity individuals still possess, and therapists should not assume that patients are incapable of any decision-making. Where a patient has only marginally or partially impaired cognitive functioning, the practitioner should seek to involve that person as far as possible in any treatment decision. If, for example, a patient is aphasic following a stroke, the practitioner should attempt to provide information in a way that the patient can understand, using pictures and simple words to communicate.

Where patients are totally unable to participate in decision-making, treatment can be given which the therapist, together with the carer, thinks is in the patient's best interests, provided the patient does not actively object. A carer, for example, could use available funding to organise for an adult with learning disabilities, living in institutionalised care, to receive CAM treatment. A therapist could lawfully provide any treatment which she felt to be in the patient's best interests.

Where the patient's condition makes it impossible to gain consent, practitioners should nonetheless work only when the patient does not object to the treatment and appears to be content for the treatment to proceed. This is generally referred to as *assent* to treatment. Patients' carers are probably best placed to shed light on the incompetent patient's preferences, although it is debatable whether someone who has lost their capacity is the same person they were before, with the same preferences. As an example, if a patient who, prior to her stroke, disliked personal contact now seems to derive immense pleasure from reflexology it would be unethical to withhold treatment because she would have rejected it in the past.

A question that arises in the treatment of mentally incapacitated patients and children is whether CAM, to the extent that it depends on patient participation, will work as effectively in either group as could be expected if the patient were a competent adult. The argument is that mentally incapacitated patients and children cannot be expected to exercise self-responsibility in the same way as rational, competent adults. If, however, CAM is shown to be successful in either group, does this mean that active patient participation is not as important as many therapists claim?

The answer may lie in what it means for the patient to be an active participant. In conventional health care ethics, this would usually be taken to mean that the patient exercises rational judgement in choosing the therapy and makes informed decisions on the basis of information given. Active participation usually refers to active participation in decision-making, rather than to the therapy itself. Making patients active participants in surgery does not mean expecting them to assist in their own operations. Rather it presupposes active deliberation about whether to agree to accept treatment.

Patient participation or active patient involvement may mean something rather different in CAM. To the extent that CAM therapists believe in the body's innate ability to heal itself, patient participation, in the sense of stimulating self-healing, does not necessarily presuppose active, volitional engagement on the part of the patient. Lack of ability to make rational, autonomous decision is no bar to the body healing itself.

Notes

1 Barton, C. and Douglas, G. (1995) *Law and Parenthood*. Butterworths: London, Dublin and Edinburgh.
2 Neeley, G.S. (1988) 'Legal and Ethical Dilemmas Surrounding Prayer as a Method of Alternative Healing for Children'. In Humber, J. and Almeder, R. (eds) *Alternative Medicine and Ethics*. Humana Press: Totowa, NJ.
3 Ibid., 174–175.
4 In the UK, this is achieved through a 'specific issue' order under section 8 of the Children Act 1989. See, for example, *Re R (A Minor) (Blood Transfusion)* [1993] 2 FLR 757 and *Re O (A Minor) (Medical Treatment)*[1993] 2 FLR, in which parental refusal of blood products was overturned.
5 Bridgeman, J. (1988) 'Because We Care? The Medical Treatment of Children'. In Sheldon, S. and Thomson, M. (eds) *Feminist Perspectives on Health Care Law*. Cavendish: London and Sydney.
6 Conroy, S., *et al.* (2000) 'Survey of Unlicensed and Off Label Drug Use in Paediatric Wards in European Countries'. *British Medical Journal*. 320: 79–82.
7 See, for example, Mill, J.S. (1859) *On Liberty*. Chapter IV. Reprinted (1974) Pelican Books: London.

17

ISSUES RELATED TO JUSTICE

Key ethical issues
* The need to demonstrate accountability
* Understanding why patients complain
* Viewing complaints as an opportunity to improve quality

As with other ethical issues previously discussed, justice is an area which individual therapists do not see as having a great deal to do with their own practice. There may be a number of reasons why this is the case.

* Since many therapists do not perceive their therapy to be intrinsically harmful, they are unlikely to make provision for things going wrong.
* The vast majority of therapists operate wholly in the private sector, with clients paying for treatment out of their own pockets. Although some therapists do operate a sliding scale of fees, few therapists involve themselves in the wider question of distributive justice. The principle of equal access demands that if CAM has the potential to benefit than it should be equally available to all and not just to people who can afford to pay for it.
* Justice is perceived as something external to the therapist. Sloppy practitioners are sometimes viewed by their peers as unlucky for being caught rather than as unprofessional. Practitioners tend not to regard commitment to the principles of justice as the responsibility of the individual.
* The comparative absence of litigation against CAM practitioners may produce a false sense of security, whereby therapists do not think of themselves so much as above the law, but rather that the law has little to do with them. Similarly, the lack of teeth of many professional bodies means that many practitioners do not think that they will be dealt with harshly even if a patient makes a formal complaint.

Accountability

The move towards professionalisation has increased practitioners' awareness of professional accountability. Accountability is an aspect of the ethical requirement to act justly and fairly. To be accountable for one's actions means being prepared to justify them and to take responsibility for their consequences. Professionals are accountable to their clients, their profession, and ultimately, to themselves. In practical terms, being accountable requires practitioners to be able to justify why they acted in a particular way. Since mechanisms for ensuring accountability operate retrospectively, clear, contemporaneous patient records are vital if the practitioner is to remember what action was taken, or what was said and why, and to have a written record as proof. Patient records may be used in evidence in any disciplinary proceedings and practitioners should always make a particular note of any area of disagreement or conflict.

Accountability is a key component of professional regulation. Whilst professional education and training hopefully minimises the likelihood of harm occurring in the first place, procedures must exist to deal with situations when something does go wrong. Most professional bodies have some form of disciplinary mechanism to deal with allegations of professional misconduct. Few CAM professions operate a separate complaints mechanism, although CAM practitioners who work in an integrated setting will be subject to the organisation's complaints mechanisms as well as those of their own professional body. Complaints mechanisms are designed primarily to protect the public, but are also important in protecting the name of the profession.

Disciplinary and complaints mechanisms should be designed to respond constructively and swiftly when an adverse incident has occurred. The credibility of a professional body will depend largely on the way in which it deals with patients' complaints about practitioner's conduct. A professional body which is consistently 'soft on its own' may find its right to self-regulate being questioned. Nonetheless, professional bodies have a duty to act justly and fairly to both practitioners and patients in exercising their disciplinary functions. Because of their quasi-public function, disciplinary procedures are amenable to judicial review and must act in accordance with natural justice. Disciplinary panels should be properly constituted with an appropriate balance of professional and lay members at all stages of disciplinary hearings. Each party must have the right to be heard and to be legally represented, if appropriate. Because the practitioner's right to practice and earn a living is at stake, there should be an independent appeal process.

Most disciplinary bodies have a range of penalties at their disposal, from a verbal or written warning at one end of the spectrum, through to de-registration at the other end. The more serious the allegation, the stronger the proof needed to convict. Rules governing disciplinary procedures need to strike an appropriate balance between formality and informality.[1] Larger professional associations tend to adopt a legalistic approach, while smaller organisations may lack the resources to convene formal proceedings. Whereas professional misconduct proceedings tend to resemble a criminal trial, complaints proceedings may be more informal and involve mediation and conciliation.

Because most disciplinary bodies require the criminal burden of proof to establish serious professional misconduct, very few cases result in practitioners having their licence to practise revoked. Self-regulatory bodies have been the subject of intense criticism for setting the standard of serious professional misconduct too high. This means that a practitioner whose performance is persistently sub-standard may not be disciplined. One response would be to lower the burden of proof from the criminal standard – *beyond reasonable doubt* – to the civil standard – *proof on a balance of probabilities*. Some regulatory bodies have responded to this by invoking a second raft of disciplinary procedures to deal with professional performance as distinct from one-off examples of serious professional misconduct. Separate procedures tend to be in place to deal with practitioners whose professional performance is seriously impaired through ill health. Practitioners have an ethical duty to ensure that poor physical or mental health does not adversely affect a patient.

Statutory regulation is thought to provide greater protection to the public than voluntary self-regulation because it involves protection of title. This means it is a criminal offence for a de-registered practitioner to continue to use their professional title, which, it is hoped, will limit their ability to practise. But, de-registration is meaningless if a practitioner can simply join another professional association and continue to treat patients. Professional associations might consider reciprocal enforcement of disciplinary findings, although this may be hard to apply across national and international borders.

Disciplinary mechanisms will only protect the public if they are sufficiently visible and accessible. Many patients do not even know what a practitioner's professional body is called, far less that they can institute a complaint. Many professional bodies rely on *ad hoc* disciplinary mechanisms which deprive both the complainant and the practitioner of access to natural justice. It is not much comfort for professional bodies to say that they hardly ever have to remove a practitioner from their register if this is because of deficiencies in the system. Since not all practitioners even belong to a professional body, it is important to consider not just how complaints are dealt with at a collective disciplinary level, but how the individual therapist can respond to patient dissatisfactions.

Learning from complaints

As the ethics of the marketplace has crept into the health care arena, patients have been recast as consumers. This has, in turn, made patients

more consumerist and more prepared to assert their rights if they are dissatisfied with the level of service they have received. Although this has had the
unfortunate effect of making some health care practitioners work defensively, in general, there has been a positive shift in the way that complaints
are perceived. Whereas in the past complaints were unwelcome and treated
defensively, a more constructive view of complaints is to see them as an
opportunity to learn from mistakes and to improve services. In a dramatic
overhaul of complaints procedures in the UK, the following principles were
identified as crucial to any effective complaints system:[2]

- responsiveness;
- quality enhancement;
- cost effectiveness;
- accessibility;
- impartiality;
- simplicity;
- speed;
- confidentiality;
- accountability.

The above criteria would certainly be necessary attributes of an organisational or collective response to complaints. In practice, it may be difficult for
CAM professional bodies to continue to combine regulatory functions and
trade union functions. In effect, the same professional body which operates
disciplinary functions may be trying to provide practitioners with support in
the event of a complaint being made against them. An independent
complaints system is more likely to allow impartiality and fairness.

In practice, many complainants are still reluctant to bring a complaint
and find complex mechanisms daunting. Wherever possible, complaints
should be handled at a local level, if possible between the individual practitioner and patient. In order for practitioners to respond appropriately to
aggrieved patients they need to gain some understanding as to why patients
complain.

Understanding why patients complain

Most practitioners set out to have healthy, constructive relationships with
their patients. Few practitioners intend to cause their patients harm or
distress. This being the case, it is vital to try to understand what motivates
patients to complain. Provided they have been appropriately informed, most
patients ought to accept that therapy cannot promise an instant cure, and
must appreciate that there are risks inherent in any form of treatment.
Patients are entitled to assume that their health will not be made worse as a
consequence of treatment, that they will be treated in a professional manner

at all times, and that their practitioner will act with courtesy and sensitivity towards them at all times.

Complaints do not simply arise because something has gone wrong. Most complaints occur because of the way that an episode has been handled. Most research in this area has identified poor communication as the biggest single factor in why people complain. Poor communication leads to unresolved conflicts, which are more likely to escalate into a formal complaint to the practitioner's professional body. Patients rarely pursue a formal complaint out of retribution or a desire for compensation. Usually, patients want an *explanation* of what has gone wrong and *reassurance* that the same thing will not happen again, either to them or to other patients. Where harm has been caused, most patients expect an *apology*. The accountability of professionals is closely linked to their visibility. Health care practitioners who work in hospitals or group settings are less able to cover over their mistakes or stifle patient's dissatisfactions. CAM practitioners, as discussed, often work in sole private practice. A consequence of this is that they are not constantly kept in check through interaction with other health practitioners. In some cases, this may lead practitioners to overestimate their own capabilities and to trivialise patients' complaints.

Practical responses to receiving a complaint

The relatively small number of complaints against practitioners suggests that most practitioners try to do the best for their patients and are committed to providing a quality service. Most practitioners are fully aware of the need to take whatever steps are necessary to protect their patients from harm. On rare occasions when a serious mistake does occur, conscientious practitioners are likely to be angry and disheartened with themselves and disappointed at letting their client down. Regrettably, not all practitioners respond to errors in their practice in the most rational way. Sometimes, the anger that practitioners feel towards themselves will be projected on to the client, with practitioners subconsciously or overtly blaming the client and exculpating themselves from blame.

Few practitioners are able to view a complaint in a positive light and may initially become defensive and regard the complainant with hostility. Although understandable, neither of these responses is constructive, since an initial conciliatory response may stop a complaint in its tracks. Whether working as a sole practitioner or as a member of a group practice, therapists need to have a complaints procedure in place, should a patient wish to complain. Within a group setting, a complaints manager should be appointed, who will be the first point of contact. Practitioners who receive a complaint might consider taking the following steps:

- If possible, diffuse the situation by receiving the complaint attentively and making the client feel assured that they are being heard. If the complaint is a reasonable one, apologise and try and ascertain how the patient can be appeased. Ask whether the patient is satisfied with a verbal apology or would feel happier if their fees were refunded. Realise that an apology does not constitute an admission of liability and may well stop the situation from spiralling.

- If the complaint or allegation is of a more serious nature and the patient is threatening to take the matter further, do not respond to the client immediately, beyond a recognition that you are taking the complaint very seriously. Tempers are likely to be running high and although there may be a desire to retaliate, this is only likely to make matters worse and may escalate the situation into a disciplinary complaint or even legal action.

- Never abuse the patient for making a complaint. This is counter-therapeutic and unprofessional.

- Write an account as soon as possible recording what was alleged by the client and what response was made.

- Elicit the views of a supervisor or mentor, if applicable. Supervisors and mentors are removed from the situation and are likely to be more objective. Do not discuss the matter with more people than is absolutely necessary and remember to preserve the patient's confidentiality when discussing the matter.

- Contact your professional organisation or defence organisation for advice.

- Depending on the nature and severity of the complaint, contact professional indemnity insurers.

Encouraging complaints

Although it may seem like taking the commitment to justice a step too far, as an ethical ideal, individual practitioners should encourage patients to voice their dissatisfactions with any aspect of the therapeutic encounter. This may require actively *facilitating* patient complaints. Practitioners can do this by displaying their professional code of ethics in the waiting room and by having a notice up outlining their complaints procedure. Professional associations should respond to complaints by patients in a constructive and supportive manner, and should have trained staff to explain to members of the public how to invoke disciplinary proceedings where necessary. Making a complaint can require a lot of courage, particularly if professional abuse is involved. Complainants must be assured that their complaint will be treated as confidential.

Complaints about other practitioners

Sometimes, when seeing new clients, it may become obvious that they have serious grounds for complaint against a practitioner they have seen previously. What should therapists do in this situation? Do they have an obligation to report another practitioner's conduct? Some practitioners might feel that this has nothing to do with them, and if the patient does not want to take the matter further, that they should not intervene. They may, with justification, feel that they have only heard the patient's side of the story and might not wish to cast aspersions on that basis. Fewer practitioners still would wish to pass judgement on the technical competencies of another practitioner. Nonetheless, there may be clear-cut situations where the practitioner is morally obliged to act. An example might be where a patient reveals that the practitioner had sex with her, saying that this was part of the therapy. It is increasingly recognised that practitioners have positive duties to protect patients from harmful colleagues. Whereas in the past, practitioners could themselves be subject to disciplinary mechanisms for disparaging a colleague, most codes of ethics require practitioners to report colleagues to the professional body where their behaviour or ill-health places patient safety at risk. Professionals who fail to report unsafe or unethical conduct may themselves be charged with serious professional misconduct.

Notes

1 See Palmer Barnes, F. (1998) *Complaints and Grievances in Psychotherapy. A Handbook of Ethical Practice*. Routledge: London and New York.
2 Department of Health (1994) '*Being Heard – The Report of a Review Committee on National Health Service Complaints Procedures* (The Wilson Report). DoH: London.

Part III

ETHICS IN PRACTICE

Introduction

Comparing groups of therapies

Even though CAM embraces a great variety of therapeutic approaches and modalities, when we concentrate on the *ethical requirements* of practitioners there is greater commonality between various therapists than there is difference. Rather than attempting to describe the ethical issues which arise in every existing therapy, Part III will look at the ethics which apply to groups of therapies which share a common approach. This is not merely to avoid the repetition of discussing, say, the need for confidentiality, in two hundred therapies. For the purpose of ethical analysis, it seems appropriate to consider these categories as giving rise to distinct ethical issues which do not apply equally to all therapies.

The six categories which will be used for ethical analysis are as follows:

Hands-on therapies: Examples include chiropractic, osteopathy, shiatsu, massage, rolfing, reflexology, aromatherapy, therapeutic touch.
Invasive therapies: Examples include acupuncture, colonic irrigation, chelation therapy and any other therapy which utilises invasive techniques.
Product-based therapies: Examples include homoeopathy, herbalism (western and Traditional Chinese herbal medicine), Ayurveda, Unani, aromatherapy, nutritional therapy, Bach flower remedies.
Energy-based medicine: Examples include spiritual healing, intercessory prayer, crystal healing, radionics, channelling, Reiki, therapeutic touch, acupuncture, shiatsu, tai chi and Qi Gong.
Psychological interventions: Examples include hypnotherapy, counselling and psychotherapy.
Self-help techniques: Examples include yoga, biofeedback, meditation, visualisation, self-hypnosis, relaxation techniques, Alexander technique, Tai Chi, Qi Gong and autogenic training.

Any attempt to categorise groups of diverse therapies will be problematic and some therapists will no doubt disagree with the classification proposed. This categorisation is based not on therapeutic approach, but on the *distinct ethical issues* raised by different categories of therapies. Any given therapy may fall within several of the categories described, for example, therapeutic touch falls within both the hand-on therapies and energy-based medicine. Similarly, acupuncture is both an invasive procedure and an energy-based approach. Therapists must decide for themselves which categories best apply to their work.

The nature of this exercise means that seemingly diverse therapies may be placed in the same category. Therapeutic touch practitioners and chiropractors may be surprised to find themselves placed side by side, but they are united to the extent that lawyers and ethicists single out the slightest 'unwanted touching' as an area for concern. Similarly, different therapies within a given category may give rise to discernible ethical differences. For example, product based-therapies have many similarities giving rise to joint ethical concerns, but also some interesting differences, such as the willingness of homoeopaths to withhold the nature of the remedy they are prescribing compared with other product-based therapists.

Use of more familiar taxonomies, such as 'whole systems' of medicine, will be avoided, since whole systems can also be assimilated into one or more of the categories below. From an ethical perspective there may be important distinctions between homoeopathy on the one hand, and acupuncture on the other. Even though both may be termed 'whole disciplines', fewer concerns are levelled against homoeopathy than acupuncture, since medical practitioners tend to be dismissive that homoeopathy can have any specific effect. Similarly a separate category of 'diagnostic techniques' (such as kinesiology, iridology or vega testing) has been avoided, because the ethical issues raised are not sufficiently distinct from other therapies, and the main ethical issues they raise, such as recognising limits of competence, have been discussed elsewhere.

The categories are not intended to be definitive. Other characteristics could justify further groupings, for example, therapies (often indigenous) whose basis for therapeutic claims rests on long usage, rather than modern scientific investigation. Nor is it intended that these categories be seen as totally distinct. Similar tensions and concerns may arise in several groups and the boundaries between groups are porous, not fixed. The groups discussed here will hopefully prompt other scholars to further define and analyse ethical tensions. As a starting point, the categories chosen reflect the ethical issues which seem to cause most anxiety to CAM practitioners and users.

18

HANDS-ON THERAPIES

Introduction

This category spans a diverse range of therapies including osteopathy, chiropractic, massage in its various forms, aromatherapy, reflexology and therapeutic touch. From an ethical standpoint, the implications of touch on people's lives cannot be understated. Many therapies seek to harness the therapeutic powers of touch.

Central to western concepts of autonomy is the notion of bodily sovereignty. A major element of controlling one's life is deciding what will happen to one's body. This involves two separate notions. The first is that individuals should be free from unwarranted interference with their bodies (for example, nobody should receive a massage unless they want one), and the second is that competent adults should be allowed to do whatever they like with their own bodies, provided it doesn't hurt anyone else. Examples might include tattooing and bungee jumping. In common law jurisdictions, there are a few exceptions to this second category. Adults are required to wear seat belts when they are driving. Such exceptions are rare, and the intrusion to personal freedom has to be justified on the basis of public safety.

This commitment to bodily integrity is recognised by the law, which creates, in many jurisdictions, an offence of touching any person without their consent. In law, trespass (otherwise known as assault or battery) recognises the inviolability of a person's body. A therapist who touches a patient without their permission may be sued in battery, even if they caused the patient no harm. The law prioritises physical harm over emotional harm, in that in order to quantify harm, the law finds it easier to work within the confines of the material body. Physical harm is an obvious risk where manipulation is involved, although some hands-on therapies will involve greater risks of harm than others. For these reasons, consent to touching is a primary concern.

As well as the right not to be touched, respect for autonomy also implies respect for the individual's privacy and dignity. This means that a patient's body should not be touched unless the patient consents. Accordingly, boundary issues are also highly relevant to this group of therapists. The appropriateness of touch varies hugely from one culture to another and therapists working in a hands-on fashion must be aware of their patient's cultural sensibilities.

Disclosure of risks and informed consent

In US and UK law, the amount of information that a practitioner needs to disclose is, broadly speaking, governed by the amount of information that a reasonable patient would wish to know in order to make an informed decision. This includes information about what the procedure involves, what its likely effects will be and any material risks involved in the procedure. The ability of a practitioner to give adequate information will depend, in part, on that information being available to the therapist. This may be derived through formal research or it may be information derived from the practitioner's personal experience, or a combination of the two. The level of information is usually determined by the perceived level of risk inherent in a therapy. Risks need to be disclosed if they are reasonably likely to materialise, or if they are less likely to occur but present a risk of reasonably serious harm. Ideally, in patient-centred practice, the practitioner should tailor the amount of information to that sought by the patient.

Risks of harm

Given the range of therapies included under this heading, it is not surprising that the risks inherent in the various hands-on therapies varies greatly. Therapies which include high-velocity manipulations have far greater capacity to cause harm than therapies which use no more than light finger pressure to achieve their therapeutic effect. Where a therapy has known risks of harm, these ought to be discussed with patients before the therapist starts. When we are discussing the risks inherent in hands-on therapies, we automatically think of physical risks first. But we must also remember that harm need not be physical harm. Any therapist may cause a patient psychological harm, for example, by imposing ill-informed, psychotherapeutic interpretations on the patient's condition.

Chiropractic and osteopathy might need to be singled out as posing particular risks to the patient. Although the incidence of complaints or legal action is extremely low, chiropractic and osteopathy, by virtue of the techniques used, carry a number of risks, ranging from relatively mild to fatal. These include:

- soft tissue injuries;
- sprains;
- fractures;

- damage to the spinal cord;
- death.

Most of these risks are limited to occur in chiropractic and osteopathy, but other hands-on therapies, such as sports massage, may also cause soft tissue injury and sprains. Additionally, any massage-based therapy may cause harm when the patient suffers from certain medical conditions in which aggressive massage may be particularly dangerous. Any practitioner using hands-on techniques should therefore be aware of the contraindications to massage. Horrigan lists extensive contraindications for use of massage, including:

- contagious disease or acute infection;
- acute undiagnosed back pain;
- respiratory insufficiency;
- deep vein thrombosis;
- varicose veins/phlebitis;
- unexplained lumps and bumps;
- low platelet count and other causes of easy bruising;
- unstable pregnancy;
- cancer patients;
- some dermatology patients;
- patients suffering from dementia and psychosis.[1]

Reflexology, although perceived as a gentle form of therapy, involving light pressure on areas of the foot, similarly has various contraindications for use. These have been listed by Griffiths as including:

- some individuals may find the intensity of this therapy unacceptable;
- reflexology is not generally used for diagnosis, except in preventive health care;
- for some conditions, for example, diabetes and hyper/hypothyroidism, the reflexologist must work closely with medical colleagues;
- reflexology is not suitable for the first trimester of pregnancy;
- reflexology should be used cautiously with patients in depressive and manic states;
- reflexology should be used with care in patients with epilepsy and in acute conditions.[2]

In all cases, practitioners should advise patients of material risks, which are those risks which a reasonably prudent patient would take into account when deciding whether or not to submit to treatment. Practitioners should take care to address the specific concerns of individual patients.

An anxious patient is complaining of persistent pain in her lower back. She submits happily to the initial examination but as soon as she lies down on the couch she tells you that she doesn't mind what you do to her provided you don't 'click her back'. You are reasonably confident that one high velocity thrust is all that will be required to substantially alleviate her symptoms and so you begin the treatment with massage and stretching techniques. When you feel that the patient is completely relaxed you perform the high velocity thrust and a loud click ensues. The patient is horrified. She leaps of the table, bashing her knee as she does so, and pulls her clothes on as she screams at you that you have betrayed her trust and that she'll never trust a chiropractor again.

In this case, the chiropractor is attempting to benefit the patient, not to undermine her wishes. Nonetheless, he has acted paternalistically in thinking that he knows better than the patient and has caused her harm by virtue of overriding her wishes. The chiropractor might have argued that his decision to perform this manoeuvre was based on his prediction of the likely outcome, namely that he anticipated that the treatment would be successful and that the patient would not mind having had her autonomy overridden for the sake of her longer term health benefits. This is an example of how difficult it can be to base moral actions on unknown future consequences. Because the chiropractor did precisely what the patient forbade him to do, the patient may be able to instigate a complaint to the practitioner's disciplinary body. His actions may also amount to the civil wrong of trespass to the person (battery).

Training requirements

The competencies required for the safe performance of hands-on therapies may be easier to pin down than in other categories. Interventions which are targeted at the material body may be easier to capture and break down into components than interventions which operate at a subtle energy level. This is not to suggest that the competencies required for hands-on therapies can be described fully by a set of rigid competencies. Even if one attempts to describe the more humanistic requirements that ethical practice requires, these will be interpreted by different therapists in different ways.

The level of training required to allow the practitioner to work in a safe, unsupervised capacity will usually relate to the capacity of the therapy to cause harm. Courses for therapeutic touch are likely to be considerably shorter therefore than the training to become a chiropractor. The level of medical knowledge included in the curriculum will also differ from therapy to therapy. This will feed into the practitioner's ability to make medical diagnoses and to share a common discourse with doctors (given the predominance of the scientific paradigm).

Different jurisdictions require different levels of training for different hands-on therapists. The *laissez-faire* regulatory stance of the UK is rather unique in this regard. Under UK common law, anyone enjoys a freedom to practise unless the therapy is statutorily regulated. At the time of writing, only osteopaths and chiropractors are statutorily regulated in this way. In the UK and elsewhere, the most invasive hands-on therapies are usually taught by three- or four-year degree courses, followed by a period of provisional professional registration and/or supervised practice. There is greater variation of training amongst the less harmful hands-on therapies, such as massage, and these therapies also tend to be less tightly regulated. A common core ethical requirement for all hands-on therapists is that they have sufficient competence to treat the particular patient and that they are aware of the limits of their competence.

Research using private patients

Most hands-on therapies would agree that safe, beneficent practice requires there to be a research base. A greater emphasis is therefore being placed on research-based practice in the more professionalised therapies. What distinct problems does research present for hands-on therapies?

A problem besetting CAM as a whole is finding enough patients (outside a hospital setting) to recruit as research subjects. A particular problem for potential researchers is how to reconcile the desire to conduct research with the fact that most patients pay for their therapy and would want to receive established treatments, rather than be guinea pigs for experimental procedures (which may or may not prove to be as good as, or better than the best available treatment). The traditional ethical view is that patients should not be coerced into acting as a research subject by either moral blackmail or monetary inducements. This is why ethics committees reject protocols where research subjects will be offered free treatment/payment-in-kind. For this reason, it would probably be ethically unacceptable to waive the fees of patients who agree to participate in trials as this might constitute an inducement.

The argument, however, that fee-paying patients should not be allowed to participate in research may not be sustainable in the long term. In the UK, it is thought to be more ethically acceptable to recruit NHS patients since they are receiving care free at the point of delivery (indeed the process of mandatory ethical review is limited to consideration of NHS patients). The issue cannot turn on treatment being 'free', for whilst NHS patients do not pay for their care directly, most pay for treatment indirectly through taxation and national insurance. Patients do not then, in some intangible way, owe the NHS a duty to participate in research because they are getting 'something for nothing'. If there is a duty to participate in research it can only be grounded in broader communitarian arguments that since we all, as citizens, stand to gain from research, we all have a civic duty to participate in research. This argument is less plausible given the extent to which research priorities are dominated by economic interests.

Two possible solutions are suggested as ways of recruiting research subjects. The first would be to recruit, where possible, from training clinics, where patients usually receive treatment from a supervised student for a reduced fee, and might be happy to participate in research in return. In the same way as most patients now accept that teaching hospitals are centres of teaching *and* research, it would be logical to extend this idea to CAM training institutions. The second solution would be to accept that if we want to recruit research subjects, we may have to start paying for their time and effort. Who will pay and whether payment would necessarily render a subject's participation unethical are questions which require further consideration.

Neither solution minimises the centrality of ensuring that patients recruited into a CAM trial have given a genuinely informed consent to participate in research. Provided patients are informed of the risks, understand what participation involves, and are not coerced, there is no reason why they should be excluded from CAM research. A corollary of this position though is that the research trials should be of a good design and be capable of yielding valuable information, otherwise it would be an abuse of the research subject's goodwill and participation for them to be involved in the research project.

Sensitivity of working with vulnerable groups

The specific and non-specific benefits of touch make hands-on therapy a useful tool in the treatment of certain groups of vulnerable patients. The traditional understanding of vulnerability refers to patients who are unable to give a legally binding consent on their own behalf. For the current purposes, it is worth adding to this group those patients who might be able to consent as a matter of law, but who are unduly dependent on the therapy and the therapist at that point in their lives, and who thus may make less than rational choices. Patients who are recovering from an addiction may fall into this category. The intimate nature of hands-on treatment means that it must be used with particular care on vulnerable patients, particularly those who are emotionally fragile or suffering from a psychiatric condition. This may be particularly relevant where the therapy is aimed at enhancing the patient's self-image, for example, using massage therapy in the treatment of patients suffering from eating disorders.

Hands-on therapies are also increasingly used in two categories of patients who cannot give consent in law, namely unconscious patients and babies. Reflexology and therapeutic touch have both been used on comatose patients and cranial osteopathy and paediatric osteopathy are both used on very small babies. The absence of consent does not mean that either of these examples are ethically unacceptable, but emphasise the need for the practitioner to have a good reason for believing that the therapy is in the patient's best interests. Unlike competent adult patients who have the freedom to choose this therapy from the range of therapies available, the incompetent patient cannot make such a choice. Accordingly, it is for the therapist to be sure that this intervention is in the patient's best interests. *This may require knowledge about other therapeutic interventions which may be of more value to the patient.* Currently, there is little research evidence to facilitate such choices.

Specific ethical issues raised by specialisation within osteopathy

Unlike many other CAM therapies, osteopathy has a number of recognised specialised areas of practice. These include: cranial osteopathy, paediatric osteopathy, sports injuries, veterinary osteopathy, and obstetrics and gynaecology. In the UK, these are usually taught as part of a post-graduate course or module of a higher degree. Specialisation and sub-specialisation goes hand in hand with a reductionist approach to health and may, increasingly, occur in hands-on therapies. As an ethical issue, the development, or extension, of a knowledge base in these areas begs the question of whether an osteopath who has *not* developed an expertise in these areas should treat patients who could benefit from treatment given by a more specialised practitioner. This is a particularly problematic question given that most hands-on practitioners tend to think that they can always do something to benefit the patient. This issue will affect any hands-on therapy as specialisation begins to occur.

Specific ethical issues raised by therapeutic massage

Massage embraces a wide variety of touch-based therapies. Massage has historic precedents, with both the Bible and the Koran referring to anointing the skin with oil.[3] Historically Japanese and Middle Eastern cultures used massage as part of their health and hygiene rituals. However, the ascendancy of the Church has curtailed the use of massage, equating physical pleasure with sin. This prurient approach has ensured that in the UK and elsewhere, massage has gained ground as a therapeutic professional, intervention in the relatively recent past. The ongoing association of therapeutic massage with massage for relaxation or sexual gratification is ethically and professionally problematic, especially given that many of the benefits of massage are due to non-specific effects and are common to all forms of massage. As is the case within aromatherapy, the onus is on therapeutically inclined practitioners to justify how, and in what way, they are offering a *clinical* treatment, as distinct from a form of relaxation. Developing the existing research base would be a possible starting point.

You are completing a three-year massage course and need to write up thirty clinical case studies. Accordingly, you are practising on whoever you can get your hands on! You are delighted to be approached by a friend of a friend, who says that he gets a lot of tension from working at a computer all day and he will happily serve as a case study. Your only previous encounter with this prospective client was at a New Year's party and your memory of that encounter is rather blurred. During the third and final therapeutic encounter, it becomes obvious that the client is highly sexually aroused and makes a sexual pass at you. You, similarly, find the client attractive, but need to finish the massage in order to be able to include this person as one of your case studies.

In a situation such as this, it would be unethical for the practitioner to continue to treat. Patients, as well as practitioners, have a responsibility to maintain boundaries, although the position is slightly less categoric here unless the student has made it sufficiently clear that this is a professional, and not a social, encounter. Practitioners must appreciate, however, that it may be extremely difficult for some patients to respect boundaries and that it is entirely *their* responsibility to make it clear what is and what is not acceptable. A brave student might nonetheless include the client as a case study, using what happened as an opportunity to reflect on how to maintain boundaries in professional relationships.

Notes

1   Horrigan, C. (1995) 'Massage;. In Rankin-Box, D. (ed.) *The Nurses' Handbook of Complementary Therapies*. Churchill Livingstone: Edinburgh.
2   Griffiths, P. (1995) 'Reflexology'. In Rankin-Box, D., op. cit.
3   See Horrigan, op. cit.

19

INVASIVE THERAPIES

Very few therapies fall into this category, which implies more than a patient being given a remedy which they will ingest. By invasive therapies, I am referring to therapies in which the therapist performs an invasive procedure on the patient's body. Examples of therapies in this category include acupuncture, colonic irrigation and chelation therapy. The points made in this section might apply equally to therapists (including hands-on/manipulative therapists), who perform invasive procedures as part of their diagnosis, for example, a chiropractor performing a rectal examination in order to assess the positioning of the coccyx.

The need for a specific category to consider invasive therapies (or invasive therapeutic techniques) is that these are most likely to harm a patient if performed by unskilled practitioners. The harm may be physical, particularly in the case of acupuncture, or may be psychological, particularly when intimate touching is involved. As the avoidance of harm is a primary ethical requirement, these therapies require particular attention. Since acupuncture is the quintessential example of an invasive therapy, it is appropriate to concentrate much of the discussion in this section on the ethical issues raised in acupuncture. The parallel is the amount of attention devoted to the ethics of surgery in mainstream bioethics. In each case, there is fascination with the power to do good in the right hands and to do harm in the wrong hands.

Acupuncture

Risks associated with acupuncture

Acupuncture embraces a wide variety of therapeutic approaches. There is considerable variation as to how it should be performed and what works best. Areas of contention include:

• the optimal location of acupuncture needles;
• the kinds of conditions which can be treated with acupuncture;

- the use of set acupuncture points rather than individual prescribing;
- the value of electro-stimulation of needles.[1]

An extensive survey of adverse effects was conducted by Rampes and James who reviewed all English language papers between 1966 and 1993. The adverse effects they identified included pneumothorax, hepatitis, spinal cord injury, septicaemia, retained needles, drowsiness, bruising and burns (from use of moxibustion).[2] As can be seen, these complications range from relatively trivial to exceedingly serious. Nonetheless, the total of 216 serious incidences occurred over a twenty-year period. In view of the millions of acupuncture encounters each year, this figure is very reassuring. In response to reports of adverse effects due to infection, most practitioners now use disposable needles. A recent report on acupuncture produced by the British Medical Association confirms that the likelihood of a patient suffering an adverse reaction from acupuncture is small, especially in comparison to the risks of conventional medicine. The report notes:

> Due to a lack of surveillance systems and standardised reporting procedures, the incidence of adverse reactions to acupuncture is difficult to assess, although one study of acupuncture (Umlauf, 1988) over a period of 10 years in a Czechoslovakian hospital evaluated 139,988 acupuncture treatments and found 8.9% (approximately 12,459 treatments) resulted in adverse events (faintness, fainting, haematoma, pneumothorax and retained needles). Considering that the Medicines Control Agency receives approximately 17,000–18,000 UK reports of suspected adverse reactions to all medicines each year, of which 55% are serious and 3% are fatal (Hansard, 2000), the incidence of adverse reactions to acupuncture appears relatively low.[3]

What is interesting from an ethical point is that none of these complications would have been caused by a *competent* acupuncturist. The adverse affects of acupuncture are *not* inherent in the therapy itself. What this demands from an ethical perspective is that all acupuncturists are sufficiently trained so that adverse events do not occur.

The form that acupuncture training ought to take is controversial, with traditional practitioners favouring a stronger traditional oriental input, and non-traditional, western acupuncturists favouring a more medicalised training. All traditional forms of acupuncture are based on the Daoist theory of yin and yang. Illness is seen as resulting from a deficiency or excess of various endogenous or exogenous factors, and treatment is aimed at restoring harmony. Unlike traditional acupuncture, most western medical acupuncturists do not treat on this basis. Acupuncture points are thought to correspond to physiological and anatomical features, and diagnosis is made in conventional terms. Treatment in western acupuncture is orientated towards providing symptomatic relief.[4] Whereas a traditional training takes several years, some doctors and physiotherapists learn to apply a limited range of points in as many months.

As a therapy which is both invasive and a whole system, there are stronger grounds for insisting that an acupuncture education equips an acupuncturist to make a differential diagnosis and to recognise when the patient has a serious medical condition. Arguably, this requirement should extend equally to all practitioners working within a 'whole system', where important issues around limits of competence and appropriate limits of the therapy itself must always be borne in mind. Drawing on the available evidence, Vincent and Furnham assert that:

> In practice, most acupuncturists recognize that many disorders do not respond to acupuncture and that acupuncture should be some-times only given as a supplement to orthodox treatment.[5]

A research base for acupuncture and Traditional Chinese Medicine

Advocates of acupuncture are keen to point out that in terms of safety and efficacy, Traditional Chinese Medicine (TCM) has been practised for several thousand years. The earliest recorded history of TCM appeared in 1800 BC at the start of the Shang dynasty. More significantly, the 'Internal Classic' or 'Yellow Emperor's Internal Classic', which dates back to 300 BC, contains the basic theory of TCM which is still used today.[6] As Saks points out, though:

> its effectiveness cannot be simply inferred from the long history of its usage in China ... for many therapies have been discredited after being practised for centuries – as, for example, bloodletting and other heroic therapies in the last century in Britain.[7]

Even a history of safe usage over time may not satisfy questions of comparative efficacy required by modern consumers to make optimal choices. The accumulation of empirical evidence over centuries does, however, provide acupuncturists with sufficient parameters to provide benef-icent treatment and to know how to avoid causing harm.

What should patients be told?

A lay person's perception of acupuncture is that it involves sticking needles into certain parts of the body to bring about a cure. Some might know that the purpose of the needles is to stimulate energy flow along meridians. If asked what conditions acupuncture treats, people would probably be able to list pain relief and might possibly cite the treatment of addictions. Whilst none of these is incorrect, the lack of knowledge that most people have about the different types of acupuncture commonly practised and the philosophical underpinnings of traditional Chinese acupuncture mean that practitioners will probably have to convey a significant amount of information about what is involved if the patient is to be an active participant in this form of therapy.

In order to respect autonomy, patients need to be told how the therapy will make them feel, as well as receive information about more serious risks. Acupuncturists need to tell patients about side effects of treatment, including possible fainting, drowsiness and bruising. Since receiving acupuncture can be daunting at first, the practitioner should be reassuring and explain what he or she is doing to the patient throughout the treatment.

There has been little discussion as to how far acupuncturists should attempt to explain to patients the philosophy underlying their practice. The Chinese understanding of health and disease is radically different from a western, biomedical interpretation. Much of the information upon which the acupuncturist is basing the treatment will mean little to the patient, unless the patient has a rudimentary understanding of chi, yin and yang, interior and exterior, etc. Without some understanding of what the practitioner is doing and why, the patient may be forced into the position of being a passive recipient of treatment, rather than an active participant in their own healing process. Acupuncturists might argue that it is possible for a patient to respond to acupuncture and for the body to begin to heal itself without the intervention of the patient's rational thought processes.

> You are a traditionally trained Chinese herbalist and you pride yourself on good communication skills. You have been treating a new client suffering chronic fatigue for several weeks. You are amazed and extremely hurt that at the end of the client's fifth visit, she says that she doesn't think you know what you are doing and she is sick of your 'half-baked theories about her heavy heart and dampness', most of which information, she claims, is a rehash of information she has given you herself. She doesn't think the therapy is helping and does not want to continue the therapeutic relationship.

This situation could have been avoided if the acupuncturist had made some attempt to describe traditional diagnosis and treatment in a way which was intelligible to a complete lay person. Better communication might have helped avoid unrealistic expectations, especially if the practitioner informed the patient at the outset that the effects of the treatment might be subtle and take some time to take effect.

Who decides which symptoms should be treated?

One issue which acupuncturists may not even have identified as an ethical matter is whether they or the patient should determine which symptoms get treated and in what order. Ideally, in a therapeutic partnership, this should be a matter for discussion. In reality, the therapist might have a very firm feeling as to which of the patient's presenting symptoms should be prioritised.

Often, an acupuncturist might feel that the patient's presenting symptoms are masking a quite different underlying health problem. Various scenarios may potentially give rise to ethical difficulties. One example would be where the practitioner disregards the patient's perception of what should be dealt with as a priority. This might be because the practitioner feels that it is more appropriate to deal with the underlying constitutional issue, otherwise the symptoms will only be temporarily resolved. Another situation would be when the patient is receiving treatment for one set of problems, but the practitioner feels that this treatment cannot proceed if there is an exterior condition which needs to be treated first.

> An acupuncturist is providing treatment for a patient's menstrual symptoms. After a few sessions, the acupuncturist feels that he has to concentrate for two sessions on treating the patient's cold, which presents as an exterior condition. Although this may make sense to the acupuncturist, the patient, had she been asked, may have preferred to take an over-the-counter remedy than to pay for two acupuncture sessions which were not directed at the longer term goal of alleviating her menstrual problems.

Conversely, practitioners may feel that they are being put on the spot by a patient who insists treatment be given in a way which runs counter to the therapist's preferences. As Fulder writes:

> For example, many acupuncturists find themselves called on to focus on symptoms more directly at the expense of the slower restoration of energetic balance, because of the expectations of patients who are conditioned by modern medicine to expect a fast restoration of comfort.[8]

These issues are not unique to acupuncture, and manifest in therapies such as homoeopathy and herbalism as well, but are more acute in a therapy where the patient may be less able to challenge what the practitioner is doing and why.

Who should provide acupuncture?

Given the safety concerns over incompetently performed acupuncture, it is reasonable to ask who should provide acupuncture. Traditional Chinese acupuncturists study both the philosophy and practice of acupuncture for several years. Increasingly though, much acupuncture is provided by medical acupuncturists, physiotherapists or CAM therapists trained in another modality (particularly osteopaths and naturopaths) who use acupuncture occasionally as a supplement to their primary therapy. Few of these providers of acupuncture have anything like as extensive a training as TCM acupuncturists. Are these practitioners responsible for a higher proportion of the adverse events? Do they pose a risk to the public? Inevitably there is disagreement on this point. Fully trained acupuncturists might feel that the acupuncture offered by practitioners who receive a diploma after a short course, or the use, by physiotherapists, of a limited number of points to provide symptomatic relief, bears no resemblance to their work and should not be called acupuncture. Medial acupuncturists, in contrast, believe that they are competent to use a more limited form of acupuncture to provide symptomatic relief.

The World Health Organisation has expressed the opinion that at this stage biomedical theory does not serve as an adequate basis for the practice of acupuncture:

> In recent decades, the theoretical and practical aspects of acupuncture have been developed in various countries, particularly in those where modern Western medical perspectives and research methodologies have been applied to studies of the traditional therapy. The achievements of these studies should be included in the training. However, since a new theoretical system has not yet been established, traditional Chinese medical theory is still taken as the basis of the Core Syllabus.[9]

Nonetheless, many doctors provide acupuncture treatment on the basis of a training which falls short of that recommended by the WHO and are resistant to the idea that they require several hundred hours of training in Oriental acupuncture before being qualified to provide acupuncture. In order that patients can make an informed choice, practitioners should provide details of their training and theoretical approach prior to treatment.

Is acupuncture patient-centred?

All acupuncturists would like to think that they practise in a patient-centred way. Earlier parts of the book have questioned whether 'patient-centred practice' necessarily involves eliciting active, volitional patient participation. In other therapies, most history-taking involves direct questioning of the patient (who is rightly deemed to be the expert in terms of his or her own body). In acupuncture, much of the information on which acupuncturists base their treatment is gleaned from pulse-taking and other observations. The actual treatment, in which the acupuncturist inserts the needles, is far more of a 'doing to' activity than a therapeutic alliance. Unless a patient is highly informed about acupuncture, it would be unusual to consult them as to where the needles should be situated. Similarly, the acupuncturist alone will decide when the needles have been in place long enough to have their desired effect (subject to them causing the patient pain and needing to be adjusted or removed).

Therapeutically, this need not defeat the suggestion that the acupuncture is patient-centred, or that the therapeutic encounter is one-sided, since the insertion of the needles will be stimulating the body to correct its imbalances and redirect energy as appropriate. This merely highlights another paradigmatic difference, namely that when CAM therapists talk about patient participation, this need not mean volitional, active involvement in the sense that conventional doctors might talk about patients exercising self-responsibility. In the absence of the mind-body dualism which characterises modern medicine, it is possible for the patient to be bringing about change at a physical level, without willing it as such. This has dramatic implications for consent, which presupposes the ability of patients to make rational decisions (that is, with their heads not their bodies) as a precursor to treatment. This deeply theoretical question is probably of less practical importance than the reality that failure adequately to inform may result in the practitioner being sued and that information should be given on this basis regardless.

Colonic irrigation

Colonic irrigation (CI) involves using apparatus to insert a high volume of water or other liquid into the colon, a few pints at a time, in order to flush out its contents. This is thought to exert a beneficial, detoxifying effect. There is little clinical evidence to support the claims made by colonic therapists. A 1995 position paper from the US National Council Against Health Fraud (NCAHF) is highly critical of CI, stating:

Colonics is popular as a health fetish. The ideas of 'cleansing' and 'detoxification' have no physiological significance, but these do have emotional meaning to people who believe themselves to be 'unclean' or 'impure' in some way. Just as the ancient Egyptians did, health neurotics may temporarily relieve their health anxieties by colonics, laxatives, and purges. Colonics also has erotic appeal to some. A substantial amount of colonic product marketing is aimed at male homosexuals. Colonics is often done in massage parlors that serve erotic desires. Colonics can be a kind of 'Dr. Feelgood quackery' (i.e., a procedure that elicits a feeling in a patient which is interpreted as beneficial).

What is interesting here is that the reasons given as to why people are attracted to this procedure pick up on many of the themes we have discussed earlier in this book. Certainly, people's usage of CI does not appear to be based on an evaluation of the available clinical evidence. People seek out CAM therapies for a variety of motives, not all of them 'health-related' in the strictest sense. This need not challenge the validity of these therapies, merely question the likelihood of their being integrated alongside more orthodox 'health' approaches.

Risks of colonic irrigation

Although not commonly included in discussions of high-risk therapy, dangers of CI may include:

* severe cramps and pains;
* removal of healthy bacteria from gut;
* death due to severe electrolyte imbalance;
* perforation of the intestinal wall;
* cross-infection from inadequately cleaned equipment.[10]

Should people be free to practise and use colonic irrigation?

CI is a useful therapy to test the limits of a government's commitment to free choice. The question is whether competent adults should be free to pursue interventions of limited medical benefit and potential serious side effects? Much turns on the nature of claims made by colonic practitioners. To the extent that practitioners make unsubstantiated medical claims, patients may have some redress through legal mechanisms. Medical licensing boards may consider use of CI by their members as a disciplinary matter.

But should practitioners be prevented from telling prospective clients that this therapy will give them a feeling of 'lightness' or 'inner well-being' if this is what clients have subjectively experienced? How 'medical' do the benefits have to be before something can be considered a *legitimate* alternative therapy (or is the phrase an oxymoron?) Should doctors be the final arbiters of what constitutes a health benefit? If we allow this to be a medical question, then we should not be surprised to learn that something becomes a health issue often when a drug or technology is developed to 'treat' it. The development of 'lifestyle' drugs, such as Viagra, is a good case in point. Even if it is felt that CI does not offer medical benefit, should people not be allowed to take bodily risks in the same way that they engage in dangerous sports, eat junk food and use licit drugs such as alcohol and tobacco?

Chelation therapy

Chelation therapy is used as an alternative treatment for chronic heart disease and peripheral vascular disease, and has been promoted as an anti-ageing technique. The procedure, used widely in the USA, involves the use of chelation (E.D.T.A, ethylenediamine tetra-acetic acid) in treating arteriosclerotic heart disease. Chelation therapy is used in the treatment of heavy metal (such as lead) poisoning. When injected into the blood, EDTA binds the metals and allow them to be removed from the body in the urine.

Side effects of chelation therapy can include cardiac arrhythmia, clotting disorders, kidney disturbance, thrombophlebitis and embolism. The use of this technique in the treatment of heart disease has been discredited by the American Heart Association, which says that there is no scientific evidence to demonstrate any benefit from this form of therapy. Concerns are expressed that reliance upon this form of unproven treatment may deprive patients of well-established benefits from the many other valuable methods of treating these coronary heart diseases. Critics of CAM will often assert that deterring a patient from seeking orthodox medical treatment which might be of more benefit is ethically unacceptable.

The ethical interest is that although there is no systematic evidence to show that this therapy is efficacious, the fact that chelation therapy is practised *by doctors* places it, for the most part, above scrutiny. If chelation therapy is, indeed, regarded as 'something doctors do', the side effects of this intervention are given less attention by the media and regulatory authorities than the side effects of CAM therapies. The contrast, in this regard, with acupuncture, is quite striking. Whereas chelation therapy is both invasive and has the potential to cause serious side effects, it is generally perceived as being less risky than acupuncture, even though acupuncture has much evidence demonstrating its effectiveness, is far less invasive, and has few reported adverse incidents.

The inclusion of chelation therapy in this section is to highlight the inherent bias against CAM practitioners performing anything more than minimally invasive therapies and the freedom, in contrast, of doctors to carry out highly risky procedures which are not of proven safety or efficacy. Within conventional medicine, it is accepted that many interventions carry risks of serious side effects, chemotherapy being an obvious example. These are thought to be justified by the potential benefits the treatment may offer. What is important, however, is that in orthodox medicine, a high level of risk is thought to be acceptable, even when the chance of a successful outcome is small. The same approach does not seem to be extended to CAM, even though the risks of CAM therapies tend to be proportionally smaller.

Notes

1   See Saks, M. (1995) *Professions and the Public Interest. Medical Power, Altruism and Alternative Medicine.* Routledge: London and New York, Chapter 4.

2   Rampes, H. and James, R. (1995) 'Complications of Acupuncture'. *Acupuncture in Medicine.* 13 (1): 26–33. Discussed in Vincent, C. and Furnham, A. (1997) *Complementary Medicine, A Research Perspective.* John Wiley & Sons: Chichester.

3   British Medical Association (2000) *Acupuncture: Efficacy, Safety and Effectiveness.* Harwood Academic Publishers: Australia and the United Kingdom. Citing Umlauf, R. (1988) 'Analysis of the Main Results of the Activity of the Acupuncture Department of Faculty Hospital'. *Acupuncture in Medicine.* 5: 16–18.

4   Vickers, A. and Zollman, C. (1999) 'ABC of Complementary Medicine. Acupuncture'. *British Medical Journal.* 319: 973–976.

5   Vincent, C and Furnham, A., op. cit.

6   Discussed in greater detail by Pei, W. (1983) 'Traditional Chinese Medicine'. In Bannerman, R., Burton, J. and Ch'en, W.C. (eds). *Traditional Medicine and Health Care Coverage.* World Health Organisation: Geneva.

7   Saks, M., op. cit.

8   Fulder, S. (1988) 'The Basic Concepts of Alternative Medicine and Their Impact on our Views of Health'. *The Journal of Alternative and Complementary Medicine.* 4(2): 147–158.

9   World Health Organisation (1999) 'Guidelines on Basic Training and Safety in Acupuncture'. Available at: http://whqlibdoc.who.int/hq/1999/WHO_EDM_TRM_99.1.pdf.

10 See, for example, Eisele, J.W. and Reay, D.T. (1980) 'Deaths Related to Coffee Enemas', *Journal of the American Medical Association.* 244: 1608–1609; Istre, G.R. *et al.* (1982) 'An Outbreak of Amebiasis Spread by Colonic Irrigation at a Chiropractic Clinic'. *New England Journal of Medicine,* 307: 339–342; Ernst, E. (1997) 'Colonic Irrigation and the Theory of Autointoxication: A Triumph of Ignorance Over Science'. *Journal of Clinical Gastroenterology.* 24:1 96–198.

20

PRODUCT-BASED THERAPIES

Examples include homoeopathy, herbalism (western and Traditional Chinese Herbal Medicine (TCHM)), Ayurveda, Unani, aromatherapy, nutritional medicine and flower remedies. As with the previous categories, the linking together of highly professionalised therapies with less well-established therapies may cause some consternation. However, our present inquiry is concerned with the areas that make this group of therapies ethically interesting and not whether ephedra is more dangerous than 'Rescue Remedy'.

A significant concern is over the regulatory status of non-conventional therapeutic products. The alternative health products market is a multi-billion dollar industry. Herbal remedies, homoeopathic remedies, aromatherapy oils, vitamins and nutritional supplements have become so mainstream that in many countries they are sold through supermarket chains. However, the regulatory status of these products occupies a dubious status between foods and medicines. Because few plant-based remedies are licensed as medicines, manufacturers are prohibited from providing information about potential health benefits, appropriate dosages or possible side effects. This position is untenable, given that these products are clearly bought by people who hope that they will be of benefit to their health.

The regulatory status of herbal medicines and herbal practitioners is particularly problematic. In the majority of EU member states, including France, Spain and Portugal, the prescribing of medicines is unlawful other than by a registered medical practitioner. In the UK, anyone may call themselves a herbalist. The status of herbal remedies in the UK relies on a historic exception to the 1968 Medicines Act, which has been repeatedly challenged. Under the current law, there are still potential risks to patients. Although patients cannot access the most toxic herbs other than through a herbalist, the absence of statutory regulation means that practitioners using the title 'herbalist' may be inadequately trained to prescribe potentially dangerous herbs such as lily of the valley (*Convallaria majalis*) or deadly nightshade (*Atropa belladonna*). The former contains substances which, in excess, could cause heart failure in those with chronic heart disease. The latter is a poison at all but therapeutic doses.

In January 2000, the Irish government withdrew the over-the-counter availability of St John's wort, notwithstanding the many studies highlighting its usefulness in treating mild to moderate depression. The rationale for its removal, along with other herbs, including *Gingko biloba, Caulophyllum thalictroides* and *Harpogophytum procumbens* was that these products clearly fell within the EU definition of medicines. Article 1 of EU Directive 65/65 EEC (European Union Council Directive 1965) defines a medicinal product as:

> Any substance or combination of substances presented for treating or preventing disease in human beings or animals. Any substance or combination of substances which may be administered to human beings or animals with a view to making a diagnosis or to restoring, correcting, or modifying physiological functions in human beings or animals is likewise considered a medicinal product.

In the UK, exemptions apply under section 12 of the Medicines Act 1968 which allow aromatherapists and herbalists to make, sell and supply remedies in the course of their business. They may also sell or supply remedies which have been manufactured for them by the holder of an appropriate manufacturing licence. Regulation 3(1) of the Medicines (Advertising) Regulations SI 1994/1932 provides that no person shall issue an advertisement relating to a medicinal product in respect of which no product licence is in force. Many manufacturers flout these provisions, making health claims for their products.[1] Legally, any claim that a product can cure, treat or prevent a disease is generally regarded as a medicinal claim, and should only be made where the product has a medicinal licence.

The problem is that in order to become licensed as a medicine, manufacturers need to demonstrate the safety, quality and efficacy of their product. Many natural remedy manufacturers have argued that they cannot afford the large-scale clinical trials needed to provide this sort of information. Herbalists argue that the complex modes of action of plant remedies are not yet fully understood, making it hard to adduce the sort of efficacy data required by licensing authorities. The inability to patent a plant/plant remedy, as compared with synthetic drugs, significantly decreases the commercial viability of investing in long-term clinical trials. The existing option, which is to describe these herbal and nutritional products as foods (which only have to demonstrate safety and quality and not efficacy), is equally unsatisfactory.

The European Pharmaceutical Committee is currently seeking a better regulatory solution.[2] Other countries have been more proactive in this regard. In Australia, for example, the government's revised Therapeutic Goods Administration allows for the recognition of non-conventional remedies and the licensing system takes account of the differences between plant remedies and synthetic drugs.

Ethical issues arising out of various product-based therapies

Aromatherapy

The Aromatherapy Organisations Council (AOC) in the UK is keen to stress the difference between clinical practitioners and beauty practitioners and defines an aromatherapist as:

> A person who has been trained to a defined standard in the use of essential oils for therapeutic purposes. An Aromatherapist may also utilise oils for beauty treatment purposes, but a person trained only in their application for beauty purposes is not considered to be an Aromatherapist.[3]

Contraindications for use

Although most essential oils are safe if used correctly, there are certain situations in which oils may cause harm. Since so many people buy their oils over-the-counter, it is important that this information comes into the public domain.

- If essential oils are combined with massage, the contraindications for massage apply.
- Essential oils must be diluted before applying to the skin.
- Sensitive patients or those with allergies should be treated with caution.
- Toxicity and contraindications for each oil must be well understood.
- In pregnancy, many oils are contraindicated due to toxic risk to mother and fetus or risk of spontaneous abortion.
- A few oils are toxic and are not recommended for general use.
- Practitioners should avoid using oils that elicit a negative psychological response from the patient by asking them about their preferences.
- Due to the strong association that smell can have with memory, special care should be taken with patients undergoing chemotherapy or those feeling very unwell and sensitive; the smell of an oil present at an uncomfortable time could, in a subsequent context, induce nausea or negative emotions.

Use of aromatherapy during pregnancy and childbirth

Aromatherapy can be beneficial during pregnancy and childbirth, and most oils are thought to be safe to use. However, some oils should be avoided or used with caution during this period. Oral administration of essential oils is thought to be particularly risky and the internal use of oils is a rare form of treatment in the UK, requiring additional training and special insurance.[4]

Tisserand identifies the following oils as having a degree of risk in pregnancy:[5]

Oils to be avoided in pregnancy	Oils to be used with caution
Camphor	Cangerana
Hyssop	Lavandula stoechas
Indian dill	Lavender cotton
Parsley leaf	Oakmoss
Parsley Seed	Rue
Spanish Sage	Treemoss
Savin	

Use of aromatherapy by nurses

Along with therapeutic touch and reflexology, aromatherapy is particularly popular with nurses. However, unless specifically negotiated, it is unlikely that use of CAM therapies fall within the nurse's usual scope of employment. This places the nurse in a potentially vulnerable position, and may conflict with her ethical, professional and legal responsibilities.

> An experienced nurse has undergone training in therapeutic touch and aromatherapy in her spare time. She has been using these therapies in private practice for ten years. She has also been using these therapies to good effect in a group of her hospital patients recovering from a stroke. Because she thinks that these therapies do not have any side effects, she has given these therapies without consent. When the relatives of one patient find this out and make a formal complaint, the nurse is disciplined by her employers for providing unconventional treatment without the hospital's permission and for treating without the patient's consent.

Any nurse intending to offer aromatherapy must ensure that her training is sufficient to enable her to work as an autonomous practitioner in this regard. A training course which spans several weekends is unlikely to satisfy this condition. A nurse who intends to incorporate therapeutic interventions should only do so with the support, and in the full knowledge of, her line manager, preferably in accordance with an established and agreed protocol. Failure to do so could result in the nurse being subject to disciplinary action by her employers or professional body.

In the UK, the nurses' professional body, the United Kingdom Central Council for Nursing, Midwifery and Health Visiting (UKCC) do not actively discourage the use of aromatherapy or other CAM techniques, but place the responsibility for doing so firmly on the individual practitioner. Their 1996 guidance states:

If a complaint is made against you, we can call you to account for any activities carried out outside conventional practice. You should carefully consider the content and status of any courses which you undertake and how you promote yourself.

Other ethical issues include ensuring that essential oils used on the wards do not interfere with the rights and comfort of the patient group as a whole, ensuring that the nurse is sufficiently competent to incorporate aromatherapy techniques, and ensuring that the introduction of aromatherapy is always in the best interests and safety of the patients and clients. At a more political level, nurses may meet resistance in trying to provide CAM therapies if these are perceived as clashing to any extent with the orthodox medicine that patients are receiving, thus nurses should always work with institutional support and knowledge.

Herbal medicine

As with many other CAM therapies, there has been a huge growth in the use of herbal medicine. Whilst herbal medicines are used by some 85 per cent of the world's population, the resurgence of natural plant remedies is even more marked in Europe, Australasia and the USA, where modern pharmaceuticals are readily available. In 1990, the value of over-the-counter (OTC) sales of plant medicines in seven EC countries was estimated at US \$2.4 billion.[6] As Newell *et al.* point out:

> It is somewhat of a paradox that at a time when there is such an unprecedented number of therapeutic drugs available for the treatment of all forms of disease, that herbal remedies continue to be demanded by the general public.[7]

The therapeutic encounter

What makes therapeutic encounters with a medical herbalist unique from an ethical standpoint is that the expectations of patients consulting a medical herbalist are probably the closest to their expectations of consulting a GP/primary care practitioner. This might impact on the therapeutic encounter in the following ways:

- patients' expectation of coming away with a remedy (as one might expect to come away from a GP with a prescription for drugs);
- the extent to which the patients might adopt a more passive role as recipients of treatment rather than as active participants in treatment choices;

- the quality of information they might reasonably expect to receive as to how the remedy will make them feel, what the likely side effects are and whether the remedy will clash with other medications they may be receiving.

The fact that patients' expectations differ from those of the practitioners deserves comment, since few herbal practitioners are trained to work in a reductionist manner. Herbalists tend not to use conventional diagnostic principles. Vincent and Furnham observe that:

> Modern western herbalists use much the same terminology and concepts and many of the same diagnostic methods as orthodox medicine, but they are interested in detecting imbalance and restoring normal function rather than acting to reverse pathology.[8]

Arthritis, for example, might be attributed to 'under-functioning of a patient's system of elimination', leading to 'an accumulation of metabolic waste products'.[9]

As is the case in many other therapies, herbalists believe strongly in the ability of the body to heal itself and see themselves as supporting the vital adaptive energy of the body. Herbalists believe that plant material is more effective in restoring function if it is used in its natural, complex form, rather than modern pharmacology which isolates and synthesises the active components of plants. A patient may be given a combination of herbal remedies hoped to stimulate healing, with each remedy tailored to the individual. As such, herbal prescribing is highly individualistic.

Recognising the limitations in a 'whole' system

Herbal medicine is a whole system of health care. Along with other therapies, such as acupuncture and homoeopathy, it provides a theoretical and practical framework for treating most ailments. Whole systems are thought to present particular ethical concerns as a patient being treated by a practitioner who can 'treat everything' may be deterred from seeking more appropriate treatment elsewhere. Many herbalists acknowledge the value of conventional treatment in acute situations. But some herbalists, noticeably practitioners who have only recently graduated, would rather treat patients within the confines of their therapy. The comprehensive nature of the herbal pharmacopaeia is likely to encourage this sense of omniscience. As with all therapies, herbalists should recognise their personal limits and inexperience and also the limits of herbal medicine where an alternative approach could be of greater benefit to the patient.

Consent and information giving

Because herbal medicine involves giving active substances to patients, a key ethical issue for herbalists is giving patients adequate information to enable patients to make an informed choice when consenting to treatment. Ideally this should include information about the likely effects of treatment, the risks of treatment, the alternatives to the treatment being offered and possible interactions with other conventional and non-conventional treatments, where these are known. Herbalists might think about how much information they ought to give patients where they are combining a remedy from several herbs. Do patients need to know the precise breakdown and the risks associated with each herb used? Arguably, if a patient is to make a meaningful choice, the answer is yes, although this depends on whether a legalistic notion of consent or a broader threshold function of consent is applied.

Quality and safety of herbal remedies

The safety profile of many herbal remedies is good, particularly in comparison with pharmaceutical equivalents designed to achieve the same function. There is, however, something of a popular misconception that because herbal remedies are natural, they are safe. Some herbs (for example, aconite, gelsemium and wild lettuce) are inherently toxic and their use should be monitored by an appropriately trained herbal practitioner. Potential risks from herbal remedies include:

- inherent toxicity;
- contamination;
- substitution;
- interaction with pharmaceutical drugs;
- poor or non-existent labelling of ingredients.

Herbalists have an ethical duty to ensure the quality and safety of the herbal products they use. The principle of non-maleficence means that herbalists must ensure that the treatments they give do not harm patients. Treatment must therefore involve careful history-taking, skilful diagnosis and awareness of the possible side effects, and any individual contraindication that the patient might have towards a particular remedy. Certain herbs are harmful in certain populations. Ephedra should be avoided by patients suffering from hypertension or glaucoma, and thujone, which may induce an abortion, should never be given to pregnant women.

Quality concerns over the use of herbal remedies have been well documented, especially in relation to the use of imported traditional Chinese herbs.[10] Chinese herbal creams prescribed by practitioners for children with eczema have been found to contain powerful topical steroids.[11] Other concerns include considerable variation in the amount of active ingredients included in herbal treatments. Awareness of the possibility of interaction with conventional medications is growing.[12] Herbalists should check that patients are not taking any prescription drugs which could adversely interact with a herbal remedy, for example, ginseng may react with insulin and should not be given to diabetic patients. Herbal remedies can increase the effect of pharmaceutical drugs (for example, kava or valerian when taken with barbiturates), or interfere with their effect (for example, echinacea and zinc, both immunostimulants, should not be given at the same time as immunosupressant drugs, such as cyclosporin or corticosteroids).[13]

Patient self-responsibility

Not all incidences of harm caused through herbal remedies can be attributed to the incompetence or neglect of the herbal practitioner. Many people who suffer harm do so by acting not on the directions of a registered herbal practitioner, but through self-prescribed ingestion of herbs. The problem then is not simply better training and regulation of herbal practitioners, but the need to for consumers to be better educated so that they can make safe choices. Much reliance in the marketing of herbal remedies is placed on the idea that these remedies are natural and, by implication, free from side effects. Although labels warn patients not to exceed the stated dose, because specific health claims are not made, labels do not have to detail side effects.[14] Regulatory authorities have been slow to impose greater safeguards, meaning that consumers are still able to buy herbal preparations labelled as foodstuffs over the counter when they clearly have medicinal effects, and are being bought as such.

> *A man is advised by his nutritional therapist (who is not a trained herbalist) to try Valerian as a cure for insomnia. Because he is able to buy these pills over the counter, he assumes that they are safe and will have a mild effect. He takes the Valerian in conjunction with a prescribed barbiturate. His wife is alarmed when he has not woken up after 14 hours and calls an ambulance. The hospital confirm that these drugs should not have been taken together as the herbal remedy increases the sedative effect of the barbiturates.*

This raises the issue of whether patients should be encouraged to receive treatment only from a registered herbal practitioner, rather than attempt to self-medicate. There is something of a tension here, in that herbal medicine, along with many other CAM therapies, supports the notion of patient self-responsibility. The noted UK herbalist, Simon Mills, explains the popularity of herbal medicine as follows:

> It must surely be that plant remedies are filling a need left unprovided for in modern health care: they are safer, more accessible, and most of all they allow everyone to take charge once more of their own health care.[15]

This does not necessarily sit well with the model of patients consulting with herbal practitioners and receiving a remedy, an encounter which is not inherently patient-empowering. But given the potential side effects of herbal remedies, and the regulatory shortfall which means consumers do not perhaps have all the information they need to make a reasoned choice, there is an argument for restricting access to remedies and making them available only through appropriately skilled practitioners. Thus, Mills continues:

> While it is clear that plants are now seen as accessible and safer alternatives to synthetic drugs, it is less well known that, *in skilled hands*, they can provide a coherent and effective alternative to professional medical practice as well, that with the appropriate approaches it is possible to transform them into very powerful curative agents as well.[16] (emphasis added)

Research issues in herbal medicine

The argument is frequently made that the more individualised and less standardised the therapy, the harder it is to conduct research. It can be hard to orchestrate a randomised control trial (RCT) if every patient presenting with a given condition receives a different herbal remedy. The way in which herbal remedies are uniquely designed for the individual patient makes it very difficult to conduct herbal research which actually reflects the way in which most practitioners treat their patients. This, however, may be rather less plausible in herbalism than other highly individualised therapies, notably homoeopathy. But although herbal prescribing is largely individualised, many herbs are routinely used to treat known conditions. The use of St John's wort in patients suffering from mild to moderate depression is a good example of this, and numerous RCTs have demonstrated its efficacy. RCTs also support the use of feverfew for preventing migraine, ginger for treating nausea and vomiting, and gingko for dementia. It is also possible to carry out pragmatic studies, evaluating herbal remedies as they would be used in clinical practice. One such study found positive results for the use of Chinese herbs to treat adult and childhood eczema.[17]

As with acupuncture, many herbalists question the need for research into traditional plant remedies which have been used for thousands of years. However, whilst extensive use of herbs over a period of time may have identified the more obvious signs of toxicity there is still need for vigilance. Newell observes:

The more subtle and chronic forms of toxicity, such as carcino-
genicity, mutagenicity and hepato-toxicity, may well have been
overlooked by previous generations and it is these types, it is
argued, of toxicities that are of most concern when assessing the
safety of herbal remedies.[18]

A second argument relates to the sort of research which is being
conducted. Most therapists do not think that research is necessary to
demonstrate the efficacy of their remedies. In this regard, they are keen to
point out the long history of safe usage. Yet it is becoming apparent that
the benefits of herbal medicine, if they are to be made available to all, will
require comparisons between herbal medicines and conventional medicines.
This may be particularly relevant where a herbal remedy, such as St John's
wort, may be as effective as conventional antidepressants such as amitripty-
line, but may have fewer side effects. This information is necessary for both
purchasers and consumers if they are to make informed choices. Calls for
this sort of research have been made in relation to greater integration.
Many herbalists who do not see integration as the way ahead may reject
calls for this kind of research to be carried out. In addition to these research
questions, which will require large-scale clinical trials, the use of case
studies and adverse reporting mechanisms would be helpful to alert other
herbalists, licensing authorities and consumers to the dangers posed by
certain herbs.

Homoeopathy

The basic tenet of homoeopathy is the principle that like cures like, or 'the
law of similars'. The appropriate remedy to prescribe is that which can cause
symptoms similar to the patient's, although the remedy will be given in a
highly diluted form. Through successive dilutions, a homoeopathic remedy
is prescribed to a patient at doses so infinitesimal that the original molecule
may no longer remain. The more times a remedy is diluted the stronger it
becomes. This is known as the theory of potentisation. It is this aspect of
how homoeopathy is thought to work that renders many orthodox physicians sceptical. An e-letter in the British Medical Journal sums up these
concerns:

> The lack of a plausible biological (actually, biochemical or biophys-
> ical) modus operandi for homoeopathic treatment is not merely a
> minor irritation: it is a fundamental objection to the idea that
> homoeopathic treatments 'work', despite the results of an excellent
> trial such as the one reported by Taylor and colleagues. We know a
> very great deal about the chemistry and physics of water, including
> how it behaves at a quantum level – if this were not true then tech-

nologies such as magnetic resonance imaging would not work. In the light of this knowledge the proposition that solutions diluted beyond the Avogadro number can act in a way which is different from that of pure water are, frankly, absurd, in the most literal sense of the term.[19]

Homoeopathy is a genuinely alternative therapy in that its mechanism defies conventional scientific wisdom. Yet, laboratory studies have reported biological effects of homoeopathic medicines on animals, plants and cells. Research studies in homoeopathy which have established that the benefits of homoeopathy are not mere placebo have caused considerable consternation within the medical profession, as they throw the entire scientific paradigm into doubt.[20] No doubt in response to the threat that this poses, the integrity of homoeopathic researchers and the quality of homoeopathic research have been savagely attacked by the scientific community. In a celebrated article in the *Lancet*, doctor and homoeopath, David Reilly, asked whether the reproducibility of evidence in favour of homoeopathy was proof that homoeopathy worked or proof of the clinical trial's capacity to produce false-positive results. Either, he argued, his research demonstrated that homoeopathy did work, or, he argued, RCTs were flawed as a scientific method for investigation since they cause false-positives.[21]

Informed consent

Homoeopathic practitioners may be unable to explain to patients how their therapy works. The amount of information that they can therefore pass on to patients may be quite limited, but this need not be a bar to a legally valid consent. As in conventional medicine, informed consent requires the homoeopath to provide the patient with adequate information about the likely effects and potential risks of the proposed treatment, the patient must be sufficiently competent to make an informed choice, and the decision must be voluntary for it to be valid. If any three of these elements are missing, the consent process will be invalid, and a patient who is harmed as a result of treatment may have a legal action in trespass or in negligence, for failure to warn. Homoeopaths, unlike other groups of therapists, have been sued. How then, can homoeopaths feasibly comply with consent requirements? Voluntariness and competence to consent are relatively straightforward (although homoeopaths need to be aware of proxy consent issues when treating children). The more troublesome issue is the extent to which homoeopaths can give patients enough information for their consent to be valid. Legally, practitioners will be expected to give the patient such information as a 'reasonable homoeopath' would give. This requires homoeopaths to keep up to date with professional developments, for example, through reading relevant journals and being aware of current research. Ethically, homoeopaths who are committed to patient-centred practice should answer patients' questions fully and truthfully.

Particular questions which homoeopaths might wish to reflect on are the extent to which they will tell people that they are working holistically and what this entails. Homoeopathic prescribing draws heavily on the patient's emotional state. Indeed, sometimes, a homoeopath may prescribe a remedy based predominantly on the patient's emotional rather than physical symptom picture. This might come as something of a surprise to patients who think that they are coming to have physical problems resolved.

Respecting patient autonomy

USE OF PLACEBO REMEDIES TO MEET A PATIENT'S
DESIRE FOR A 'PILL-FOR-EVERY-ILL'

Homoeopaths have the same problem as herbalists in that many of their patients are more used to conventional consultations and conventional models of prescribing. This is an example of recognising the power of the conventional paradigm, in which patients have come to expect that when they go and see a practitioner, they will come away with either a prescription or medication to be taken there and then. This is also problematic within general practice, where patient demands have led to massive over-prescribing of antibiotics for viral infections.

Some homoeopaths deliberately resort to the use of placebos to meet the patient's desire to be given a remedy. They justify the use of a placebo on the basis that the particular patient's psychological need for a remedy is so great that healing will not occur unless a placebo is given. An example might be where the homoeopath has prescribed a remedy which is slow acting and may take two or three months to achieve its effect. Such is the desire for a quick fix that, in a case such as this, a patient may resent leaving consultations empty handed. To meet these expectations, some practitioners prescribe 'saclac' (a lactose-based dummy pill without any active remedy) to satisfy the patient that they have been given something.

This is a significant ethical issue, raising concerns about deception and paternalism. Many homoeopaths regard this as going against the whole spirit of a patient-centred relationship. As previously discussed, paternalism is not a bad thing *per se*, but it requires knowing a patient exceptionally well before the homoeopath can assert with confidence that the deception or overriding of autonomy is definitely in that particular patient's best interests. Practitioners should consider ethical alternatives, including explaining at the outset that remedies may be slow acting, because they are dealing with the root of the problem and not just the physical symptoms.

Not every patient wishes to be treated holistically. Some patients present with certain symptoms which they wish to be resolved, such as a persistent cough or a migraine, and are not interested, or are positively opposed, to the homoeopath delving any deeper. Although most homoeopaths work holistically, some homoeopathic remedies can be used symptomatically, such as arnica for bruising and trauma, cantharis for cystitis and rhus toxicodendron for joint pain.[22]

However, the aim of most classical homoeopaths is to find a single remedy which corresponds to a patient's 'constitution' and will address the underlying cause of a patient's problems, so as to prevent a recurrence of symptoms. This can be a slow process and the healing process is likely to involve a flare up of childhood symptoms.

An adult patient being treated for asthma experiences a dramatic one-off recurrence of their childhood eczema, before noticing a significant improvement in her asthma. Fortunately, the homoeopath has warned the patient about this possibility and explained that this is a sign that the remedy is working.

If a patient insists on being treated symptomatically, a homoeopath needs to explain that although it is possible to treat symptoms on this occasion, this will not resolve their problems and the symptoms will reoccur. If the patient does not want the homoeopath to proceed, the homoeopath must decide whether she is willing to treat symptomatically, and if not, whether to make a referral to another homoeopath, perhaps one who prescribes on the basis of conventional diagnosis alone.

It is not uncommon for homoeopaths to withhold the name of the remedy they are prescribing to a patient. Two main justifications are given. The first is that some homoeopaths feel that in order for the patient to be able to report back their response to a remedy in an unbiased way, they should not be told which remedy they have been prescribed, in case they go off and consult a *Materia Medica* to see what symptom profile that remedy responds to. This constitutes unwarranted paternalism and if the patient specifically asks, then withholding the name of the remedy goes against most people's understanding of patient-centred practice. In conventional medicine, the comparison would be a general practitioner writing the patient a prescription, but refusing to give any details about the drug in case it influenced the patient's response.

A second reason is that patients might be disturbed if they knew the origin of the remedy. This is particularly likely in relation to nosodes, that is, remedies made from diseased tissue.

A thirty-year-old female patient seeks treatment for non-specific urethritis (NSU). She has had a variety of problems in the pelvic region in the past. The patient is extrovert and has an active sex life. The homoeopath's remedy of choice is Medorrhinum. Because this remedy is made from the gonorrhoeal virus, she believes that it would be best not to tell the patient what remedy has been given.

In order to determine whether withholding this information is ethically acceptable, it is necessary to consider the homoeopath's motives. Homoeopaths might argue that it would be impossible to explain to a new patient, who has only a vague notion that like cures like, that in prescribing this remedy, the practitioner is not inferring that the NSU is sexually transmitted, or that the patient is the sort of patient who might get a sexually transmitted disease. Certainly, it would take time to discuss the principles underlying homoeopathic prescribing, but with effective communication skills, this should not be an insuperable task. If the homoeopath is withholding the information because she is pre-empting the patient's response and cannot be bothered to deal with the client's anger, this would not be an acceptable reason to withhold the name.

There may, however, be rare cases in which the homoeopath believes that withholding the name of the remedy will spare the patient from harm.

A forty-year-old woman has a strong fear of getting cancer. Her mother and several aunts developed cancer in their early fifties. The homoeopath withholds the fact that he has prescribed Carcinosin, a remedy made from stomach cancer cells. Even though the homoeopath is sure that this is the best remedy to give, he is sure that his patient would have a strong aversion to taking it.

This scenario would justify the homoeopath exercising his 'therapeutic privilege' to withhold information which he has reason to believe would cause the patient more harm than good. Practitioners should ensure that they only withhold information on this basis. To do otherwise would undermine the patient's autonomy.

Computer-Assisted Diagnosis – can patients help to choose their own remedy?

When, if ever, might it be appropriate for patients to assist in the choice of remedy? Most homoeopaths would insist that whereas the patient is best placed to describe their symptoms, only trained homoeopaths have the expertise to interpret and prioritise these symptoms, and to go on to select the appropriate remedy. The process by which homoeopaths arrive at their choice of remedy is shrouded in mystery, but might, in a more patient-centred model, be an area in which the patient's judgement as to priority of symptoms should be given greater weight. Before prescribing a remedy, a patient-centred practitioner could usefully say to a patient: 'On the basis of what you have told me today, I am hearing that these are the physical and emotional issues which ought to guide the choice of remedy. Do you agree?' This will allow the patient to clarify any potential misunderstandings and will make the patient more involved in the therapeutic endeavour.

Taking this idea one step further, a number of computer programs have now been designed which will match patient symptoms to appropriate remedies. Should homoeopaths encourage patients to use these themselves? Many homoeopaths would feel that this would be inappropriate, because patients lack the objectivity to self-prescribe. This may be a legitimate concern, but another reason that some practitioners may object might be because this development would constitute a threat to their livelihood. Such fears are unwarranted, because most patients derive considerable benefit from the non-specific effects of the therapeutic encounter and not just from the active component of the treatment. These issues also arises over the use of over-the-counter homoeopathic remedies and the extent to which homoeopaths feel that they can recommend these to their patients. Patient safety is the prime concern and homoeopaths must be assured that any product which they are recommending is of good quality and that patients are clear about dosage and possible side effects.

Homoeopathic research

As with herbalism, homoeopathic prescribing is highly individualised. The appropriate remedy is chosen on the basis of a detailed 'drug picture', which takes account not just of physical symptoms, but also of physical information that the patient may consider unusual (for example, whether the patient sweats more at night or during the day, whether the patient has been craving sweet or salty foods, and what weather triggers off symptoms), as well as the patient's emotions and feelings. This individualised prescribing means that two patients with seemingly identical symptoms will probably be prescribed quite different remedies. As is the case with herbalism, this has a significant bearing on homoeopathic research and the ability to conduct large-scale clinical trials of a particular remedy. Where large scale trials have been conducted, for example, an RCT for hayfever which compared homoeopathically prepared grass pollen against a placebo, they have been criticised for not representing how most homoeopaths would treat in practice. As with other individualised modalities, pragmatic studies are required to test remedies as they are used ordinarily.

Use of homoeopathy in acute medical conditions

Much of the medical profession's concern with homoeopathy is its use in acute medical conditions. There is little concern over the use of homoeopathy in non-acute or self-limiting conditions, perhaps because homoeopathy treats many of the chronic conditions for which conventional medicine has no cure. Concerns intensify, however, when homoeopaths treat patients suffering from acute medical conditions, such as sepsis or cancer. Conventional doctors argue that they, and not homoeopaths, should treat acutely ill patients. Homoeopaths disagree, arguing that they are competent to treat acute conditions, and that the clearer the symptom profile is (as in the case of sepsis or cellulitis), the quicker the patient should respond to the correct remedy. Treatment of acute conditions requires the homoeopath to intervene quickly if the remedy is not having the desired effect and to recommend urgent conventional medical treatment if necessary.

Ultimately, the choice must be the patient's, but the patient's ability to choose will depend on the extent to which homoeopaths can give patients adequate information about the benefits and risks of homoeopathy in treating an acute condition. Homoeopaths should liaise with the patient's GP/primary physician – with the patient's consent – whenever they are treating patients suffering from acute medical conditions. This is in the patient's interests as this means that there is a comprehensive record of what treatment has been given.

Treating children

Homoeopaths treat children for a wide array of conditions, including coughs, colds, earache, asthma, eczema, colic, croup and teething disorders. The law stipulates that parents of children unable to consent for themselves can agree to treatment which is in the patient's best interests. This question is especially important when contemplating treatment for children suffering from acute medical conditions, since their health can deteriorate very quickly unless they receive effective treatment. The requirement to provide treatment which is in a patient's *best interests* may put further pressure on homoeopaths to conduct comparative research, so that homoeopathic treatment can be compared with conventional medical interventions. This is particularly pressing in the case of vaccination, which some homoeopaths believe to cause more harm than good. Some lay homoeopaths offer alternatives to vaccination, such as *Pulsitilla* for measles prophylaxis, although these have not been subjected to clinical trials.

Nutritional therapy

The use of nutritional supplements has risen sharply in recent years. One hundred million Americans supplement their diets with vitamins, minerals, herbs, amino acids, or other nutritional substances.[23] Although some patients consult a nutritional therapist, many CAM therapists dispense nutritional advice as part of their attempts to make patients more responsible for their own well-being. Such practitioners may recommend certain supplements or dietary modification, along with fasting to improve health. Most of the consumption of nutritional supplements is through over-the-counter sales. Regulatory controls over nutritional supplements vary from jurisdiction to jurisdiction. In the USA, the 1994 Dietary Supplement Health and Education Act made it easier for consumers to access natural products but also loosened federal control over dietary supplements. Many indigenous dietary supplements slip through the net of formal licensing procedures (be it as a foodstuff or a medicine). Nutritional medicine may also take the form of dietary modification, in which therapists advise patients to combine various food groups or exclude certain foods from their diets (examples being the Hay diet, macrobiotics or veganism), sometimes recommending nutritional supplements in addition.

Examples of nutritional supplementation

The use of nutritional supplements is interesting ethically, because nutritional supplements are taken for very diverse conditions. As Vickers and Zollman describe, supplements are used for:

- high-dose vitamin C for cancer;
- zinc for the common cold;
- high-dose vitamins for learning disability ('orthomolecular' therapy);
- evening primrose oil for atopic dermatitis;
- evening primrose oil for pre-menstrual syndrome;
- vitamin B-6 for morning sickness;
- vitamin B-6 for pre-menstrual syndrome;
- garlic for lowering cardiovascular risk;
- multivitamins for improvement in general health.[24]

Since many patients using nutritional supplements may be seriously ill, accurate information is vital. Therapists must continue to lobby their respective governments to ensure that labelling provides information about possible benefits and appropriate dosage. The potential side effects of nutritional supplements also need to be made clearer, since many patients will assume that if a small amount of a food stuff is good for them, then a large amount will probably be better.

Integration with conventional medicine

Unlike other therapies which are practised by conventional health care practitioners as well as 'lay' therapists, nutritional medicine does not carry the widespread support of the medical profession. Dieticians, who are state-registered professionals supplementary to medicine, are sceptical of the claims made by nutritional medicine and regard the advice given in the name of 'optimum nutrition' as being highly questionable. Nutritional therapists should conduct research in their practices, for example, comparing outcomes with other practitioners. Adverse effects should always be noted and forwarded to the relevant professional journal, as these have implications for patient safety.

Nutritional advice given by non-qualified CAM therapists

One of the biggest concerns about nutritional medicine is that many CAM practitioners, will provide nutritional advice, whether or not they are qualified to do so. Most would say that dietary and nutritional advice is an integral part of treating patients holistically. Since nutritional medicine is a discipline in its own right, other CAM practitioners need to be sure that they work within the limits of their competence when providing nutritional advice, and ensure that what they recommend is based on evidence, not personal opinion.

Notes

1 The Food Commission (1997) 'Food Supplement Claims'. London. For further discussion, see Dimond, B. (1998) *The Legal Aspects of Complementary Therapy Practice*. Churchill Livingstone: Edinburgh.
2 Association Europeennedes Speccialits Pharmaceutiques Grand (1999) 'Herbal Medicine Products in the European Union. A Report'. ETD/97/336. Brussels.
3 Cited in Dimond, B., op. cit.
4 Jenkins, S. 'Aromatherapy'. Reproduced in Featherstone, C. and Forsyth, L. (1997) *Medical Marriage: The New Partnership Between Orthodox and Complementary Medicine*. Findhorn Press: Findhorn, Scotland.
5 Tisserand, R. (1995) *Essential Oil Safety*. Churchill Livingstone: Edinburgh. Table reproduced by Jenkins, op. cit.
6 Keller, K. (1994) 'Phytotherapy on the European Level'. *European Phytotelegram*. 6: 40–49.
7 Newell, C.A., Anderson, L.A. and Phillipson, J.D. (1996) *Herbal Medicines. A Guide for Health Care Professionals*. The Pharmaceutical Press: London.
8 Vincent, C. and Furnham, A. (1997) *Complementary Medicine. A Research Perspective*. John Wiley & Sons. Chichester.
9 Vickers, A. and Zollman, C. (1999) 'ABC of Complementary Medicine. Herbal Medicine'. *British Medical Journal*. 319: 1050–1053.
10 See, for example, De Smet, P.A.G.M. (ed.) *et.al.* (1992) *Adverse Effects of Herbal Drugs*. Vol. 1., Springer-Verlag: Berlin and New York; De Smet, P.A.G.M. (ed.) *et.al.* (1993) *Adverse Effects of Herbal Drugs*. Vol. 2., Springer-Verlag: Berlin and New York.
11 Harper, J. (1994) 'Traditional Chinese Medicine for Eczema'. *British Medical Journal*. 308: 489–490. More recently, a study of eleven herbal creams found eight to contain steroids: Keane, F.M., Munn, D.E., du Vivier, A.W.P., Taylor,

N.F. and Higgins, E.M. (1999) 'Analysis of Chinese Herbal Creams Prescribed for Dermatological Conditions'. *British Medical Journal*. 318: 563–564.
12 See, for example, Newell *et al.*, op. cit., Appendix 1.
13 Miller, L.G. (1998) 'Herbal Medicinals; Selected Clinical Considerations Focusing on Known or Potential Drug–Herb Interactions'. *Archives of Internal Medicine*. 158: 2200–2211.
14 Medicines Act 1968.
15 Mills, S. (1989) *The Complete Guide to Modern Herbalism*. Thorsons: London.
16 Ibid.
17 Discussed by Vickers and Zollman, op. cit.
18 Newell *et al.*, op. cit.
19 Fisken, R.A. (2000) 'The Science of Homeopathy', e letter. *British Medical Journal*. August 19.
20 Linde, K., Clausius, N., Ramirez, G., Melchart, D., Eitel, F., Hedges, LV, *et al.* (1997) 'Are the Effects of Homoeopathy Placebo Effects? A Meta-analysis of Placebo-controlled Trials'. *Lancet*. 350: 834–843.
21 Reilly, D.T., Taylor, M.A., McSharry. C. and Aitchison, T. (1986) 'Is Homoeopathy a Placebo Response? Controlled Trial of Homoeopathic Potency, With Pollen in Hayfever as Model'. *Lancet*. ii: 881–886.
22 Vickers, A. and Zollman, C. (1999) 'ABC of Complementary Medicine. Homoeopathy'. *British Medical Journal*. 319: 1115–1118.
23 Report of the Senate Committee on Labour and Human Resources on the Dietary Supplement Health and Education Act of 1994. Report 103–410, 103d Cong., 2d Sess. (Oct. 8, 1994). Cited in Cohen, M. (1998) *Complementary and Alternative Medicine: Legal Boundaries and Regulatory Perspectives*. Johns Hopkins University Press: Baltimore, MD and London.
24 Vickers, A. and Zollman, C. (1999) 'ABC of Complementary Medicine. Unconventional Approaches to Nutritional Medicine'. *British Medical Journal*. 319: 1419–1422.

21

ENERGY-BASED MEDICINE

Energy-based medicine embraces a wide range of techniques. It includes faith healing, laying-on of hands, therapeutic touch, Reiki, psychic healing, absent healing and channelling. Whereas western doctors do not accept the legitimacy of subtle energies, eastern religious and healing traditions have drawn on concepts of non-material energies such as 'prana' (life force), or 'chi' (vital energy) for thousands of years. Healing is an integral aspect of 'whole disciplines', including Ayurvedic medicine and Navajo healing. The secularisation of many western societies and the absence of spirituality in most people's lives has meant that, even within CAM, discussion about healing is marginalised.

What is healing?

The UK's Confederation of Healing Organisations defines healing as follows:

> To the extent that it occurs, healing is the transference of harmonising paraphysical energies. What energies are transferred depend on the needs, beliefs, capabilities and procedures of the persons involved. Every living being is maintained by these energies which may be transferred in the presence of those concerned or at a distance. Healing may be one individual to another or between groups and individuals or it may be self-induced.[1]

Quantifying the unquantifiable

From an ethical perspective, the most challenging aspect of the diverse range of healing practices is that they are the least amenable to measurement and quantification. Despite methodological problems, there have been many studies to determine the effects of healing. Double-blind studies have shown that healing can accelerate wound healing in mice and animals, affect enzymes, and reduce pain.[2] In a recent systematic review of randomised trials considering the efficacy of forms of distance healing (including prayer, mental healing, therapeutic touch and spiritual healing) 57 per cent of trials demonstrated a statistically significant treatment effect.[3]

Little is known about how healing works. This not only has implications for research, but also for a patient's ability to consent. Although people may agree to undergo healing, sceptics argue that this agreement cannot constitute a *rational* choice. To agree to receive the healing energy of the gods, or a higher being, cannot be conceptualised in the same way as consenting to surgery. Indeed, the challenge to rationality is one of the most important areas posed by energy-based medicine. A threshold model of consent might be all that is achievable, where the patient agrees to subject herself to the healing ministrations of another, without knowing exactly what the healing will involve or how it may work, or what its longer term affects might be.

In the holistic holy trinity of mind, body and spirit, only energy-based medicine operates predominantly in the spiritual realm. In contrast to other CAM therapies, where the practitioner has something additional to offer the patient by way of intervention, energy-based medicine is an area where the essence of the healing intervention is in the practitioner herself. Scientists who currently lack the measuring tools to detect shifts in energy might choose to attribute any healing benefit to the non-specific effects of the therapeutic intervention. The difference is that usually in energy-based medicine, these non-specific effects are the sole source of the healing activity, rather than an 'add-on extra'. Of course, it could be argued that healing therapies provide an excellent argument for challenging existing models of science, both by demanding explanations of phenomena which cannot currently be explained (for example, developing tools to measure 'energy') and also by moving the focus away from predominantly objective measures to reliance on subjective measures if no objective measures are possible.

Acquiring competence: can healing be taught?

Some healers feel that their ability to heal is a gift and that healing cannot be taught. This position is challenging to those who would insist that what cannot be taught cannot be assessed, and what cannot be assessed cannot be accredited. Again, this raises concerns that energy-based healing is unscientific because it rests on non-observable phenomena, such as intuition. This is not to suggest that healing does not require certain distinct competencies, but that it involves skills which are themselves hard to measure, or indeed, rationalise, such as transmitting the healing power of love.

As a consequence, healing requires different forms of training and induction than other therapies which more closely resemble conventional medicine. Where healing forms part of indigenous traditions, a practitioner may acquire skills through familiarisation of sacred texts and induction by elders. Writing on therapeutic touch, Egan notes that knowing when and how to use therapeutic touch requires mentorship and practice.[4] Therapeutic touch is learned through an apprenticeship. In this learning process, it may take one or two years to perfect a knowledgeable practice.

The desire to conform with the dominant scientific paradigm has seen many CAM courses adopting a modular, diploma or degree format. Whereas apprenticeships and mentorships are seen as valuable teaching methods in traditional healing systems, the training of health care practitioners in the west favours classroom-based academic training. Both students practising from a training clinic, and healers working with a mentor, need to think carefully about claims to expertise.

Particular concerns have been expressed in relation to the competence of Reiki practitioners. Reiki is taught at three levels. The first degree covers the use of hands to channel the Reiki energy, the second degree covers mental and emotional balancing and distant healing practices and the third degree enables Reiki practitioners to teach others. Although traditional Reiki trainers recommend that Reiki students wait between courses to integrate what they have learned, practitioners can legitimately call themselves a Reiki practitioner after completing the first degree, which can be taught over a weekend.[5] Although healing is not inherently harmful, practitioners should, as in all other therapeutic modalities, work within the limits of their competence.

Should healers charge for their 'gift'?

Some healers, who regard their healing powers as a gift, choose not to charge for their services. Often, healers will choose, instead, to ask patients for a donation, particularly when they are working in a religious or charitable context. This puts them at odds with other therapists who charge a fee comparable to other CAM therapies. It is not unreasonable for any therapist who has invested time in acquiring a therapeutic skill to charge an appropriate commercial rate for those services. As with all therapies, the operation of a sliding scale of fees allows practitioners to widen access to patients who would not otherwise be able to afford treatment.

Is healing more akin to religion than medicine?

There may be a significant overlap between healing and religion. Many formalised religions include a healing ministry and many healers believe that their powers come from a divine being. This can put practitioners at odds with their patients, if their patients do not believe the healing has a divine source. To this end, the Confederation of Healing Organisations' Code of Ethics specifies that to avoid offending some patients, healers must not raise the question of their religious beliefs unless this is invited by the patient.

The religious connotations of healing have interesting implications for the regulation of healing. Freedom of religion is highly valued in liberal democracies. It is not perceived to be a legitimate role of government to dictate who or what people can believe in. Attempts to interfere with religious freedom are likely to be deemed unconstitutional and an unwarranted intrusion into the private lives of citizens. By extension, belief in healing is a matter of personal choice and cannot be regulated by the government any more than religion can be regulated.

How does this apply when religious belief directly impacts upon health? The principle of respect for autonomy means allowing competent individuals to make their own choices. It does not matter whether those choices appear rational or irrational to anyone other than the patient, provided the patient has arrived at their choice voluntarily and on the basis of appropriate information. A non-believer might view the decision of a Jehovah's Witness patient to bleed to death as irrational, yet courts have upheld repeatedly the right of Jehovah's Witnesses to pursue their religious belief, even if it results in their death.

Is healing complementary to, or an alternative to, conventional medicine?

Most healers view their work as complementary to orthodox medicine. The UK's National Federation of Spiritual Healers (NFSH) describes healing in the following terms:

> Healing often helps with the speed and extent of recovery from serious illness and major surgery and from the effects of treatments such as chemotherapy and radiation therapy. It complements conventional medicine.

Healing becomes controversial when patients refuse conventional treatment either for themselves, or for their children, preferring to rely solely on healing instead. Many states in the USA have statutes which protect parents, who rely on prayer rather than medical care, from charges of child abuse and neglect. In the UK, a more pragmatic, case-by-case approach is taken. Whereas courts will ratify the decisions of adults who take decisions which may result in their own death, there is an aversion towards allowing parents to make decisions which will result in the death of their child. Courts have ordered medical treatment against the wishes of parents in a number of cases. Such decisions reveal much about the underlying antipathy towards CAM where serious illness is concerned. They also reveal deep-seated discomfort at allowing people to pursue radically alternative lifestyles. Practitioners should realise that courts will probably adopt a narrow interpretation of a child's best interests and are unlikely to look favourably upon practitioners who deliver CAM when a child would probably have benefited from conventional medical treatment.

Treating children

As therapies which bypass rational thought processes, healing can be applied to incompetent groups, such as children, or patients in a coma. Indeed, some energy-based practitioners feel that children are especially amenable to healing, because their minds offer less resistance. Nonetheless, the vulnerable status of children means that special considerations apply to healing babies and young persons who may be particularly sensitive to treatment. In relation to therapeutic touch, it is recommended that energy be given slowly and in small amounts by an experienced practitioner. Healing should only ever be performed with parental consent.

A six-year-old boy is in an intensive care unit following a road traffic accident. One of the nurses involved has developed a special interest in healing, and has started to incorporate prayer into her care of critically ill patients. Without seeking permission, she uses prayer as part of caring for this patient. When his parents are informed of this by another nurse, they are very cross, as they are both atheists and do not appreciate the nurse's intervention.

As this case demonstrates, if healing or prayer is to be used as a form of treatment, practitioners should ensure that they have the patient's consent, or obtain proxy consent from someone in a position to give it.

Use of healing without a patient's knowledge

The right to offer healing is rarely challenged. This may be because most people assume that even if healing does no good, it is unlikely to do any harm. However, when healing is intended to be used as a therapeutic intervention, all the usual patient safeguards, such as consent and confidentiality, should be present. Intercessory prayer (prayer carried out on behalf of another) cannot, of course, be prohibited by law, but clinical trials designed to measure its effects must similarly extend all the usual protections to research subjects.[6]

A trial was carried out to test the effects of remote, intercessory prayer on 999 patients newly admitted to a coronary care unit in a US hospital. On admission, patients were randomised either to receive remote prayer or not. Patients were unaware that they were being prayed for, and the intercessors did not meet the patients. The group of patients in the prayer group had better outcomes than those in the control group.[7]

The significant issue in this research is that the Research Ethics Committee approved this research even though the patients were not told that they were in a study or that they would potentially be randomised into a group receiving distance prayer. This was on the basis that there is no known harm associated with receiving remote prayer and that the process of gaining informed consent could be distressing to patients, particularly those who would wish to receive remote prayer, but who knew that they might be in the group which did not. Neither of these arguments is ethically sustainable. Well-designed studies should not prejudge the issue of whether the treatment under investigation carries risk of harm. Additionally, the distress patients might experience is precisely the reason that informed consent should have been sought. By omitting to gain consent, the researchers may have included patients who, if asked, would most definitely not have wanted to be recruited. The significant issue for therapists is that they should not agree to take part in a research study unless they are satisfied that the research subjects' rights have been met. Even when an ethics committee has approved a trial, this does not absolve individual practitioners involved in research from exercising their own accountability.

Therapeutic touch

Therapeutic touch is an interesting example of healing, in that it is practised largely by nurses. In the USA and Canada, therapeutic touch is taught at 75 schools and universities, and practised at 95 health facilities.[8] A growing number of nursing associations are interested in the application of therapeutic touch in clinical settings. Therapeutic touch is based on the assumption that a 'human energy field' extends beyond the skin. This life energy is the same as Hindu 'prana', and Chinese 'Qi' or 'chi'. Practitioners believe that this human energy field is abundant and flows in balanced patterns in health but is depleted and/or unbalanced in illness or injury. Practitioners believe they can restore health by sensing and adjusting such fields.

Dolores Krieger, who pioneered this technique, has presented anecdotal reports of therapeutic touch relieving many conditions, including premenstrual syndrome, depression, complications in premature babies, and secondary infections due to HIV. Further well-conducted research trials are necessary to evaluate some of these far-reaching claims for therapeutic touch. Nurses, working within an evidence-based climate, may find themselves put under pressure to submit the claims of therapeutic touch to clinical research, especially if they want to practise therapeutic touch within the NHS or other state-funded institutions.

Although therapeutic touch is assumed to be beneficial and free from side effects, O'Mathna is concerned that the potential harms of therapeutic touch have been downplayed.[9] There may be concerns that if the practitioner were emotionally upset or physically ill, this 'negative energy' could be transmitted to patients. Krieger herself warns that therapeutic touch practitioners must be sensitive to their client's tolerance level. She warns against flooding weakened patients with too much energy, which can overwhelm them, leading to restlessness, irritability, and anxiety that may be expressed as hostility, or felt as pain by the healee. Therapeutic touch should not be directed at the site of cancer tumours in case this makes them more, not less, virulent. Care should be taken particularly when using therapeutic touch on children, who are more sensitive and may be more likely to experience side effects.

Notes

1 College of Healing. Appendix III to the British Complementary Medicine Association (BCMA)'s Code of Conduct.
2 Benor, D.J. (1990) 'Survey of Spiritual Healing Research'. *Contemporary Medical Research*. 4(3): 9–32.
3 Astin, J.A., Harkness, E. and Ernst, E. (2000) 'The Efficacy of "Distant Healing": A Systematic Review of Randomized Trials. *Annals of Internal Medicine*. 132(11), June 6: :903–10
4 Egan, E.C. (1998) 'Therapeutic Touch'. In Snyder, M. and Lindquist, R. (eds) *Complementary Alternative Therapies in Nursing* (3rd edition). Springer Publishing Company Inc.: New York.
5 Dimond, B. (1998) *The Legal Aspects of Complementary Therapy Practice*. Churchill Livingstone: Edinburgh
6 Goldstein, J. (2000) 'Waiving Informed Consent for Research on Spiritual Matters?' *Archives of Internal Medicine*. 160, June 26.
7 Harris, W., Gowda, M., Kolb, J., Strychacz, C., Vacek, J., Jones, P., Forker, A., O'Keefe, J. and McCallister, B. (1999) 'A Randomized Control Trial of the Effects of Remote, Intercessory Prayer on Outcomes in Patients Admitted to the Coronary Care Unit'. *Archives of Internal Medicine*. 159: 2273–2278
8 Krieger, D. (1997) *Therapeutic Touch Inner Workbook: Ventures in Transperson Healing*. Santa Fe, NM: Bear & Company.
9 O'Mathna, D.P. (1998) 'Therapeutic Touch: What Could Be the Harm?' *The Scientific Review of Alternative Medicine*. Spring. Prometheus Books.

22

PSYCHOLOGICAL
INTERVENTIONS

Examples include counselling, psychotherapy and hypnotherapy. Some argue that purely psychological interventions should be excluded from discussion of CAM therapies, since psychological interventions, cannot, by definition, be holistic. I reject this argument for the same reason that energy-based medicine is included in CAM. Whilst energy-based medicine operates at a subtle energetic level, its benefits can be psychological or physiological. Similarly, psychological interventions can improve a patient's physiological and spiritual well-being. Another reason for including this category is that whether explicitly or not, most therapists draw on psychotherapeutic techniques, whatever their therapeutic discipline. It might be said that the extent to which working holistically requires consideration and probing of the patient's emotional state, a psychotherapeutic dynamic is being created, whether the therapist would describe it in those terms or not.

Counselling and psychotherapy

Psychotherapy is the systematic use of a relationship between therapist and patient – as opposed to physical or social methods – to produce changes in cognition, feelings and behaviour. Psychotherapy is a generic term covering a spectrum of treatments that can be grouped under four main headings: analytic therapy, cognitive behavioural therapy, family therapy, and creative therapies such as psychodrama and art therapy. Each of these can be brief or long term and delivered to individuals, couples, or families and groups.[1] It can be difficult for a patient to know which psychotherapeutic approach will best serve his or her needs and the evidence base for many branches of psychotherapy is slim. The lack of regulation of counselling and psychotherapy in the UK compounds these difficulties.

Most counsellors and psychotherapists deal with people who may be unhappy or dissatisfied with certain areas of their life, but who are not, for the main part, 'ill' in psychiatric terms. Were patients to exhibit signs of psychiatric illness, the counsellor or psychotherapist would have a duty to refer the patient to an appropriate medical practitioner. The parallel with CAM is important, given that a number of CAM patients are similarly not 'ill' within any conventional diagnosis, but would like to optimise their health or prevent future ill health, in much the same way as patients receiving counselling or psychotherapy may otherwise be quite pleased with the direction their life is taking, but may wish to manage a certain area of their life a bit better.

Some ethical controversies in counselling and psychotherapy

Many of the ethical issues which arise in the therapeutic relationship do so because of the dynamics of the relationship between the therapist and the patient. The effects of transference and counter-transference, discussed earlier, affect relationships between therapists and their clients, and may lead patients to have unrealistic emotional expectations of their therapists. This can lead to disappointment if the therapy fails to deliver results.

Creating dependency rather than encouraging autonomy

Most counsellors and psychotherapists regard enhancing the client's autonomy as their central goal. Enhancing individual autonomy is seen as a positive thing, as it enables the client to live their life to the full. Counselling and psychotherapy flourish in cultures in which individual autonomy is prized. Yet inherent in this objective is a paradox. In order to enhance the client's autonomy, the practitioner may deliberately, or inadvertently, foster a sense of dependence on the part of the patient. Rather than taking control of their own lives, patients may look to the therapist to supply the answers to the meaning of life and may be unwilling to take major (or minor) decisions without having discussed them in therapy first. Where patients surrender their autonomy to a therapist, the therapist must scrupulously avoid taking advantage of the patient.

Dependence on a beneficent therapist is not harmful in itself, and may be a useful and even necessary therapeutic tool. Yet, dependence within the therapeutic relationship is ethically controversial, since it relies on the paternalistic assumption that the 'therapist knows best'. A therapist would probably describe the psychotherapeutic process as providing the patient with a safe space in which to explore possible courses of action. But whereas most therapies create a temporary dependence to facilitate longer term enhanced autonomy, analytic psychotherapy, because of its indeterminate goals and indefinite length, can lead to financial exploitation in interminable therapy.[2] Holmes and Lindley warn:

[W]ithin the private sector, where fees are the subject of private negotiation between patient and therapist, there is a risk that a patient will be paying high fees over a long period without the therapy actually getting anywhere. It is possible for unscrupulous therapists to maintain this arrangement by ensuring that their patients remain permanently dependent on them. This then becomes a form of exploitation, since the therapist uses a position of relative power to take advantage of the patient.[3]

The important point to note is that any level of dependency should be explicitly recognised by the therapist as part of the therapeutic process, and be managed as such. It is also essential that patients be properly assessed before receiving psychological treatments.

A danger of CAM practitioners, as opposed to psychotherapists, utilising psychotherapeutic techniques without adequate training is that they may foster patient dependency but then be unable to encourage patients to make their own decisions. This may happen if the therapist herself becomes emotionally dependent on maintaining a particular therapeutic relationship to gratify her own unconscious needs. This may result in patients remaining in therapy for longer than is therapeutically desirable. Within counselling and psychotherapy, the likelihood of such a situation arising is minimised by professional bodies requiring therapists to be in therapy themselves. Some, but by no means all CAM therapists, receive their own psychotherapy. This is another reason why CAM therapists should seek supervision of their professional practice.

Failure to diagnose serious underlying psychological conditions

Failure to diagnose medical conditions is one of the major criticisms levelled against CAM practitioners. Physicians routinely express concern that CAM practitioners are not taught enough about conventional medicine to make a conventional diagnosis (indeed most codes of ethics explicitly prohibit CAM practitioners from making a diagnosis). The fear is that when a patient consults a CAM practitioner, he or she may remain in ignorance as to the seriousness of their condition, which neither they, nor the CAM practitioner appreciate. The pathology may go untreated and deteriorate whilst the patient pursues a complementary approach. The same issues arise in relation to a patient's psychopathology. If CAM practitioners are to use counselling or psychotherapeutic techniques, they must be sufficiently able to detect any psychiatric condition which the patient may be suffering from. Ultimately, this might not alter the course of action the therapist, or indeed the patient, decides to take, but at least the patient will be informed and be able to make better choices.

Some ethically controversial techniques in counselling and psychotherapy

Regression therapy

The history of psychiatry is littered with therapies which have subsequently been discredited as inhumane, and even barbaric.[4] The unregulated nature of counselling and psychotherapy means that many controversial therapies may still be in use, practised by inadequately trained therapists. Considerable concerns have been expressed over the use of regression therapy. The belief is that in recovering or reliving memories repressed in childhood, the patient will be able to overcome trauma and experience psychological growth. The use of these therapies has been seriously discredited following numerous allegations of 'false memories', where adult patients undergoing therapy have recovered 'memories' of child abuse, often involving a family member. The consequences of such memories have led to prosecutions of family members for incest, suicides and murder. This has led to a number of accusations of negligence against therapists in the USA, brought by third parties who have been accused of abusing clients.

> As a result of therapy for depression and bulimia, Holly Ramona, aged 24, recovered memories of sexual abuse by her father. Her therapist told her that 80 per cent of bulimic patients had been sexually abused. Consequently, Gary Ramona's wife divorced him, his three daughters broke off ties with him and he was dismissed from his job. Holly Ramona brought an action against her father. He, in turn, sued Holly's therapists, claiming they had implanted the memories of abuse. His claim was successful and he was awarded $475,000 in damages. Holly Ramona's case against her father was dismissed, on the basis that the earlier ruling established no abuse had occurred.[5]

The existence of false memory syndrome has caused considerable controversy in the medical establishment. Child abuse specialists argue that not to believe adults who claim to have been psychologically or physically abused inflicts further trauma on them. They argue that since the extent of child abuse is only now beginning to be acknowledged, it is dangerous to rule out therapeutic techniques which may help patients to remember past traumas. Others insist that reliance cannot be placed on 'recovered' memories. False memory syndrome describes the way in which memories can be created, particularly in patients vulnerable to suggestion. Several sets of guidelines now warn against the use of recovered memory techniques. A strong consequential argument against the use of these techniques is that if patients have repressed memories, it is likely to be because remembering would cause significant trauma and could affect psychological functioning. Arguably then, a therapist should avoid using these techniques if the consequences of recovery are going to cause more harm to the patient than if they remain repressed.

Rebirthing techniques

This technique was developed in the 1970s by a psychotherapist, Leonard Orr, and is a modern day variation on 'primal therapy' founded by Janov in the 1960s. In this technique, a patient is talked through the birth process. Attempts may be made to wrap up the patient to simulate the feelings experienced by a fetus during uterine contractions and birth. The therapy primarily involves a breathing technique and usually lasts no more than fifteen minutes. The practice has been banned in the US State of Colorado following the death, in 2000, of a ten-year-old girl.[6]

> *Candace N was an adopted child, diagnosed as suffering from reactive detachment disorder, a rare, but classified psychiatric disorder associated with failure to bond in infancy. Her mother paid for Candace to undergo intensive therapy sessions to improve her condition. During a rebirthing session, Candace was wrapped in a blanket secured at either end and surrounded by pillows. She was then squashed by two social workers who ran the centre and two assistants with a combined weight of 304 kg for forty minutes and taunted verbally to squeeze and push herself through to be 'reborn'. Despite her repeated cries that she could not breathe, Candace's obvious distress was ignored. When she was unwrapped after twenty minutes of silence, she was blue and suffering from oxygen deprivation. She died the following day. A post-mortem recorded asphyxiation as the cause of death. The therapists who carried out the treatment were later convicted to sixteen to forty-eight years' imprisonment. Legislation, known as Candace's Law, has been implemented to ban the use of restraint in psychotherapy.*

It is worth reflecting that in most instances rebirthing techniques do not have adverse physical side effects. This raises the question of defining and defining and standardising what this technique involves and, significantly, determining who is appropriately trained to provide it.

Hypnotherapy

The induction of a trance, or altered state of consciousness, has been used throughout the centuries to bring about health benefits across a variety of cultures. Hypnosis is used as an alternative to anaesthesia in both western and eastern traditions. Rankin-Box describes hypnosis as the conscious use of the natural trance state to provide a link with the unconscious mind through suggestion.[7] Hypnotherapy is often used as an adjunct to other psychological treatments. Once in a hypnotic trance, the hypnotherapist gives the patient therapeutic suggestions aimed at relieving symptoms or encouraging changes in behaviour. A hypnotherapist might, for example, suggest to a patient who is trying to stop smoking that the patient will no longer find smoking pleasurable. Hypnosis can be used to alleviate chronic pain by helping the patient to focus on something more pleasurable.

The main ethical concern is that a patient who is put into a trance is in an unusually vulnerable position if the hypnotherapist chooses to abuse the patient's trust and to make suggestions which are not in the patient's interests or to act in an unprofessional manner. Vickers rejects this suggestion, asserting that all hypnosis is, in fact, self-hypnosis.[8]

Nonetheless, fears about hypnotherapy have been heightened by a number of cases in which people who have been hypnotised on stage for entertainment have suffered harmful consequences, or even death. In one case, a young woman of 24 died from a fit five hours after being hypnotised in a nightclub. She had been told to emerge from a hypnotic trance as if a 10,000-volt electric shock had passed through her chair. An inquest found that she had died from natural causes, although this is being contested.[9] In another case, a patient sued a hypnotherapist for causing psychiatric harm and leading her to attempt suicide twice. This patient had also been asked to imagine that she was being brought out of her trance by an electric shock. The Hypnotism Act 1952 regulates the use of hypnotism for entertainment purposes, but does not prohibit its use for scientific or research purposes, or for the treatment of mental or physical disease.

Possible benefits of hypnotherapy

The US Agency for Health Care Policy and Research (AHCPR) reviewed various studies into chronic pain.[10] It found strong evidence supporting the evidence of hypnosis in alleviating chronic pain associated with cancer. Other data suggest that hypnosis may be effective in the treatment of irritable bowel syndrome, temporomandibular disorders and tension headaches. Hypnotherapy has also been shown to have benefits in stress management, pain control, childbirth, the treatment of phobias and the treatment of addictions.

Contraindications for using hypnotherapy

Although there are no obvious physical side effects of hypnotherapy, there are potential psychological side effects to hypnotherapy, and patients for whom use of hypnotherapy is contraindicated. Rankin-Box identifies three contraindications:

- whilst hypnosis can be extremely valuable it is important that the therapist is competent to deal with the particular problem;
- practitioners should avoid longstanding psychological problems which may require professional counselling or treatment;
- occasionally clients may feel light-headed when coming out of a deep trance state and it is important to know how to manage this and any adverse reactions that may occur.[11]

Treating children and mentally incompetent adults

Hypnotherapy requires the volition and participation of the client. As such, hypnotherapy requires that the subject be sufficiently competent to understand what the therapy involves and the possible side effects and be able to consent to being induced into a trance state. The nature of hypnotherapy means that it should be avoided in patients suffering from established or borderline psychosis and personality disorders. There may be situations in which hypnotherapy is appropriate for children, such as the use of simple trance techniques to numb an area that needs suturing, or the use of hypnosis to relieve anxiety, pain and nausea associated with cancer treatment. In such cases, hypnosis will be ethically and legally justified provided the treatment is considered to be in the child's best interests.

Notes

1 Holmes, J. (1994) 'Controversies in Management Psychotherapy – A Luxury The NHS Cannot Afford? More Expensive Not To Treat'. *British Medical Journal.* 309, 22 October 22: 1070–1071.
2 See Holmes, J. and Lindley, R. (1998) *The Values of Psychotherapy* (revised edition). Karnac Books: London.
3 Ibid.
4 Fennell, P. (1995) *Treatment Without Consent: Law, Psychiatry and the Treatment of Mentally Disordered People Since 1845.* Routledge: London and New York.
5 For further details and discussion, see Jenkins, P. (1997) *Counselling, Psychotherapy and the Law.* Sage: Thousand Oaks, CA, London and New Delhi.
6 Jofeson, D. (2001) 'Rebirthing Therapy Banned After Girl Died in 70 Minute Struggle'. *British Medical Journal.* 322, April 28: 1014.
7 Rankin-Box, D. (1995) *The Nurses' Handbook of Complementary Therapies.* Churchill Livingstone: Edinburgh.
8 Vickers, A. (1993) *Complementary Medicine and Disability: Alternatives for People with Disabling Conditions.* Chapman and Hall: London.
9 Reported in Dimond, B. (1998). *The Legal Aspects of Complementary Therapy Practice.* Churchill Livingstone: Edinburgh.
10 NIH Technology Assessment Panel on Integration of Behavioural and Relaxation Approaches into the Treatment of Chronic Pain and Insomnia (1996) 'Integration of Behavioural and Relaxation Approaches into the Treatment of Chronic Pain and Insomnia'. *Journal of the Amercian Medical Association.* 276: 313–318.
11 Rankin-Box, op. cit.

23

SELF-HELP THERAPIES

Examples include yoga, Qi Gong, Tai Chi, biofeedback, meditation, visualisation, deep breathing, muscle relaxation and self-hypnosis. For the main part, self-help techniques raise fewer ethical concerns than other CAM therapies, since the potential for the person to cause themselves harm is extremely low. Obvious ethical concerns still exist, in that practitioners who teach self-help techniques, either in a group or an individual setting, must comply with the familiar ethical imperatives, such as obtaining consent, respecting confidentiality and maintaining safe boundaries.

Yoga

The popularity of yoga has grown enormously over the last few years. Although many people have enjoyed the gentle forms of hatha and sivananda yoga, iyengar and ashtanga are currently attracting a new generation of followers. At first sight, yoga does not stand out as an activity which gives rise to ethical concerns. Yet, closer examination will reveal that yoga raises some quite unexpected issues.

Technical competence

There is a wide variety in training standards for yoga teachers. Outside India, many forms of yoga flourish. Some forms are more regulated than others and there is a great deal of variety in terms of styles, levels of intensity and training requirements. Some forms focus on relaxation and breathing, whereas others require high levels of physical strength, suppleness and concentration. Because of the kudos attached to studying under certain gurus in India, many teachers merely have to mention the guru's name to attract students, even though it is obviously very difficult to verify that someone has in fact studied under that particular guru at all.

Because yoga is commonly perceived as a leisure pursuit rather than as a form of medicine, there is not the same level of regulation of yoga teachers that one would find in areas which involve physically invasive practices. Although it might be hard, if not impossible, to regulate yoga, there is no doubt that students can cause themselves serious injury if they perform a posture, or *asana*, incorrectly. The need for expert tuition and effective supervision is, therefore, an ethical issue. However, this overlooks the fact that many people choose to practise yoga independently, in the privacy of their own home. As with the shopper who buys homoeopathic remedies in the drugstore, such individuals must exercise self-responsibility, and if they cause themselves harm, they are unlikely to find external redress.

Training

Should all yoga teachers have a formal teaching qualification or is it sufficient for a teacher merely to pass on the wisdom they have accumulated from their own teachers and gurus? The question is a dramatic example of charismatic forms of knowledge rather than externally accredited knowledge bases. As part of a religious and cultural tradition, yoga has so far managed to escape compartmentalisation into competencies which can be taught in a diploma or degree. Nonetheless, students might be alarmed to know if, for example, their teacher qualified from a teacher training course along with 200 other candidates practising at the same time, for which mere attendance and the payment of tuition fees guaranteed the acquisition of a teaching certificate.

In the sense that yoga is a form of healing tradition, the ethical issue is whether yoga teachers have a moral obligation to protect their students from harming themselves. To the extent that yoga teachers ask students at the start of a class whether they have any injuries, one would suppose that this means that they have been trained to know how to respond in that eventuality. The harms inherent in guru worship may ultimately be more serious and longer lasting than the relatively minor harm of falling out of a headstand.

Class size

The increasing popularity of yoga means that class sizes can be much larger than is ideal, with teachers attracting as many as a hundred students to a class. However much a teacher moves around during the practice, it is impossible to offer as much instruction to individual students as if one were working on a one-to-one basis. Yoga centres/individual teachers ought to restrict classes to a manageable size. Unfortunately, few centres want to turn away prospective students. Nonetheless, this is a safety issue and students with pre-existing injuries or those who need special attention are less likely to get it if there is a very full class. Unless a teacher retains a teaching space, chances are that money for classes will be collected by the centre. This minimises the likelihood of potential students observing a class, which they might reasonably wish to do before seeing whether they wish to take up yoga. Objections to observing might be that you can only get a feel for yoga through doing it, and that allowing observers may make existing students feel uncomfortable or self-conscious.

Pre-existing injuries

Particular ethical concerns are raised by teaching students who have pre-existing injuries or who are pregnant. Such students require additional expertise, and may need to have postures specially adapted for them, or ought to avoid other postures altogether. An experienced teacher ought to be able to adapt postures to accommodate the individual needs of all class members. Realistically, though, because of the way that most classes are organised, students are unlikely to be screened or refused admittance to a class. Accordingly, teachers can only minimise harm by emphasising the need for these students not to over-exert themselves.

Respecting the student's autonomy

As with all health endeavours, the student's well-being should be regarded as paramount. This can be testing for teachers, part of whose function is to push students in an encouraging fashion and help them realise their potential. Teachers should never push students, physically or emotionally, beyond the point with which the student is comfortable. This, however, is a hotly debatable area. Much of the inspiration in a yoga class may come from the teacher helping students into postures which they feel they would not be able to accomplish on their own. Both teacher and student must exercise responsibility and recognise the student's realistic limits, although this requires explicit communication and probably not just intuition.

Promoting self-responsibility

Yoga teachers believe that daily practice of postures promotes good health and enhances students' sense of well-being. Unless one is receiving 'yoga massage', no-one can do yoga practice on someone else's behalf. Essentially, yoga practice demands commitment and self-responsibility. It is important for teachers to foster a sense of self-responsibility and self-reliance in their students, particularly if class sizes prohibit individual attention. Most teachers encourage self-practice, as students will often not appreciate their strengths and weaknesses until they work through postures on their own. There is an ethical issue in how dogmatic teachers should be in relation to practice. For most westerners, yoga, along with other forms of exercise or relaxation, has to be fitted into a pressured lifestyle. Even if daily practice is ideal, it is dubious how much value there is in making students feel guilty if they can only commit to one class per week.

Emotional and physical boundaries – exploring the guru–disciple relationship

How far should teachers discourage idolisation by students? In a physical endeavour such as yoga, marvelling at one's teacher may often provide the inspiration to stretch oneself and so develop. Unfortunately, the capacity for transference and projection is significant, particularly when the activity involves adjustments which, to the uninitiated, may seem like quasi-intimate touching. Teachers can exert a considerable influence over their students' lives. What responsibilities, if any, are idolised teachers under, to prevent their students being harmed?

For the main part, few yoga students form the same level of devotional attachment to a teacher or guru as is observed and encouraged in eastern traditions. Increasingly though, fashionable yoga teachers attract a significant, and often international following. Their status sometimes transcends that of a mere teacher and assumes guru-like proportions in the eyes of their students. As the physiques of more and more celebrities are sculpted through branches of yoga such as astanga vinyasa yoga, some teachers themselves are achieving celebrity status.

Does this phenomenon have any bearing on the subject matter of this book? The focus on individual rights and freedoms in the west would tend to imply that if rational adults want to dedicate substantial proportions of their time, energy and money tying themselves in knots in pursuit of a higher self, that is their own business and not a matter which should trouble bioethicists. However, an aim of this book is to challenge orthodox ways of thinking and to expand definitions of health and well-being to accommodate the healing potential of alternative modalities. Since yoga is often included in discussions of CAM in terms of its healing potential, it seems reasonable to put the relationship between yoga teachers and their students under the microscope and to compare and contrast this relationship with that of other CAM practitioners and their patients.

It is worth noting that the full understanding of the role of the guru in Chinese, Japanese, Tibetan and other eastern cultures refers to a level of spiritual attainment and enlightenment which cannot easily be understood by many secular westerners. Within the guru–disciple relationship, there are, however, familiar comparisons with psychoanalysts and analysands. The guru is the absolute master, the wise father, who offers the path to self-enlightenment. Devotion to the teachings of the guru must be absolute, and may make considerable demands on the disciple's physical and mental energies, even requiring the complete abandonment of the disciple's previous lifestyle. Successful guru–disciple relationships have the power to transform lives and deepen a disciple's spiritual and emotional well-being. Sadly, however, the grossly distorted power differential between the two parties has repeatedly been abused and there are well-documented accounts of people's lives having been destroyed by such abusive encounters.

A moral relativist would argue that it is not appropriate for a westerner with western values to judge the rightness or wrongness of such an occurrence. When however, eastern concepts are transported into western culture and matters arise which could realistically find themselves being adjudicated within a western judicial systems based on Judaeo-Christian tradition, important cross-cultural problems arise which generate ethical questions which need to be resolved.

Ethically, we may not judge the problems raised so categorically. As people in a position of authority and power, what sorts of demands might reasonably be placed on gurus or teachers in this context? The following list of suggestions mirror previous recommendations relating to contracts and maintaining safe boundaries. As applied to yoga teachers, they make for interesting material. Requirements could include:

- yoga teachers should always work within their competence and should not teach or demonstrate postures beyond their capabilities;
- yoga teachers should not advise on health issues beyond their areas of competence (yoga);
- yoga teachers should explain their orientation and teaching method at the start of each class, so that any new student can decide whether or not this sort of class and teacher is right for them;
- where appropriate, yoga teachers should display, or be prepared to divulge, any certificates or qualifications they possess and should discuss with students what their own training requires;
- yoga teachers should avoid excessive self-disclosure;
- yoga teachers should restrict class sizes so that they may provide safe and adequate supervision of each student's practice;
- yoga teachers should discourage excessive personal gifts from students and generally refuse social invitations;
- yoga teachers should refrain from advising students on areas outside their expertise, and should be wary of unduly influencing students' personal decisions;
- yoga teachers should not allow themselves to have 'favourite' students;
- yoga teachers should refrain from intimate physical contact and should avoid entering into sexual relationships with their students.

These recommendations are similar to those contained in one of the few codes of ethics for yoga teachers, disseminated by the Association of Yoga Teachers of California. Such recommendations, which seem self-evident in relation to other CAM therapists, seem implausible and unrealistic when applied to yoga teachers. Most students would certainly not view all of the above recommendations as being of equal value. Any student who has basked in the warmth of a revered teacher's praise, or who is picked on more often than others to demonstrate a posture, would feel hypocritical in arguing that teachers should never display favouritism!

Two other responses merit consideration. It could be argued that for all its philosophical tradition as one of the great eastern religions, yoga in the west is really nothing more than a form of sport or leisure, and as such, should fall outside the realm of regulatory authorities. This has parallels with other healing traditions that have already been discussed which also lose much of their traditional flavour when re-marketed for western users. To suggest that yoga teachers should not advise on health is thus to miss the point: yoga is a whole system of spiritual, emotional and physical well-being.

Another argument against formalising the ethics of this relationship is that yoga is an example of a healing modality which requires that *the student exercise as much self-responsibility as the teacher*. Unless a western student is truly committed to renouncing western values and following the path to enlightenment, with all that it entails, the student also needs to respect and maintain appropriate boundaries, not abdicate all their autonomy by relinquishing decisions to somebody who may be very proficient at yoga, but who may not necessarily be the most enlightened personal adviser. The more the emphasis is placed on student, client or patient self-responsibility, the less the ethical analysis can rely solely on the duties of the practitioner, to the exclusion of the reciprocal responsibilities of the individual. Yoga teachers should of course act ethically, but should, at the same time, encourage their students to act likewise.

Relaxation techniques

Relaxation techniques are an integral aspect of several complementary therapies, including massage, yoga and hypnosis. They may also be used in conventional treatment, for example, as part of a behavioural therapeutic approach to pain management and insomnia. Relaxation techniques are also commonly used as a self-regulatory activity as part of stress management. The primary objective of relaxation techniques is the achievement of non-directed relaxation, rather than direct achievement of a specific therapeutic goal. Various methods may be used to induce deep or brief relaxation. Many of the following deep relaxation methods have an abbreviated form, which people can use to achieve relaxation on their own. Deep relaxation techniques include:

Autogenic training

This is a deep relaxation method which involves imagining a peaceful environment and comforting body sensations. Autogenic training concentrates on a variety of focussing techniques, including warmth or heaviness in the limbs, cardiac regulation, focussing on breathing, warmth in the upper abdomen, and coolness in the forehead.

Meditation

Meditation can either be practised on its own, or as part of another therapy, such as yoga. Meditation involves relaxing the body and stilling the mind, so as to achieve a point of non-judgemental awareness of bodily and mental sensations occurring in the present moment. The subject remains alert, but attempts to clear the mind of active thought processes. There are many forms of meditation, including transcendental meditation, in which the subject focusses on a mantra which is repeated continuously. Meditation may be combined with movement. Some forms of meditation, such as Vipassana, involve a ten-day, residential meditation, during which speech is forbidden. Such drastic meditation is not recommended for people with serious mental illnesses.

Muscle relaxation

Many practitioners make use of muscle relaxation techniques. These involve systematically tensing and then relaxing various parts of the body or groups of muscles, until the whole body is fully relaxed. In progressive muscle relaxation (PMR), all fifteen major muscle groups are tensed and then relaxed in sequence. Usually performed whilst the person is lying on the floor, a state of relaxation is maintained for ten minutes or more. Relaxation of the muscles is often co-ordinated with breath movements, with tension being released with each exhalation.

Tai Chi

The ancient Chinese practice of Tai Chi involves slow and graceful movements which are designed to improve strength, balance and mental calmness. In China and Japan, millions of people practise Tai Chi at dawn. In the UK, Tai Chi tends to be taught in classes. Similar concerns arise as in yoga, including a need to impose limits on class size, the competence of the teacher, and balancing attention to the group as a whole with attention to the specific needs of individual students.

Visualisation

A relaxed state is induced through the use of a visual suggestion. The patient will often be responsible for generating his or her own visualisation, or they may be given a prompt by the practitioner. Vickers and Zollman give the example of cancer patients being asked to think of a visual representation of their cancer cells being killed off:

> One patient might imagine immune cells as sharks and the cancer cells as small fishes being eaten; another might think of a computer game in which the cancer cells are 'zapped' by spaceships.[1]

Therapeutic benefits of relaxation

Most relaxation techniques result in decreased metabolic activity. Studies have shown that relaxation techniques can reduce anxiety, particularly during stressful situations, such as cancer treatment. As such, relaxation techniques provide a useful adjunct to conventional care. Relaxation techniques may also be useful to alleviate insomnia and panic disorders. Trials have shown Tai Chi to reduce falls and fear of falls in elderly people.[2]

Ethical issues

Self-responsibility

As self-guided activities, people need to exercise self-responsibility when utilising relaxation techniques. Although rare, some relaxation techniques may cause side effects. For example, patients who have a history of epilepsy or psychosis have experienced acute episodes after prolonged meditation.[3] A practitioner intending to induce relaxation for the first time needs to take a detailed client history and to provide information about side effects, where relevant. Even though relaxation is predominantly a self-help technique, therapists need to ensure that the subject is comfortable.

A stress management counsellor is teaching relaxation skills in a group setting, using progressive muscle relaxation techniques. To enhance relaxation, she puts on a CD of birdsong and guides the students to imagine themselves amongst the birds on a warm summer's day. Unfortunately, one student has an intense phobia about birds and finds the experience very distressing. Because all of the other students are lying down and deeply relaxed, she feels unable to say anything.

As with most CAM encounters, the patient as well as the practitioner needs to exercise self-responsibility. In the above case, the student could reasonably have requested that different background sounds be used. Practitioners should appreciate that even in such a setting, some people are uncomfortable in challenging a teacher's instructions, especially when there are other people present. Since such a situation is detrimental to the student's well-being: practitioners should always encourage students or patients to voice their concerns and not to suffer in silence.

Competence of practitioners using relaxation techniques

The competence of practitioners teaching relaxation techniques remains problematic. Practitioners need to have appropriate training to induce states of relaxation, including experience of helping people who experience emotional distress as a result of relaxation. The development of formal competencies would be useful in this area. Research into the potential usefulness of relaxation is compromised because the various relaxation techniques are not well described, there is little standardisation of therapy manuals and there is a wide variation in practitioner training. These issues will have to be addressed before relaxation techniques can be integrated into conventional health care.[4] As with all CAM therapies, reliance on relaxation techniques may deter a patient from seeking conventional treatment.

A woman has been attending weekly meditation classes to relieve the symptoms of tension headaches. Although there is some initial relief, the intensity and frequency of the headaches increases. The teacher recommends that the student uses aromatherapy oils in her bath and eliminates chocolate, red wine and citrus fruits from her diet. Several months later, medical tests reveal that the woman has a brain tumour.

As discussed, many CAM Codes of Ethics prohibit practitioners from making a medical diagnosis. In the above case, it would be unreasonable to expect that the practitioner would be in a position to diagnose a tumour, but reasonable to expect that the practitioner advises the patient to be checked over by a physician to rule out any organic basis for her headaches.

Philosophical basis for relaxation techniques

As with other traditionally based therapies, relaxation techniques may draw on eastern philosophies of energy and energy balance which are alien to western ways of thinking. However, a thorough understanding of eastern philosophies is not a prerequisite to benefiting from these techniques. Much research exists in ancient yogic and Bhuddist texts, although this will need to be built upon if relaxation is to be used as part of conventional health care. The US National Institutes for Health has called for further research comparing relaxation techniques with pharmacological treatments.[5]

Research base for relaxation techniques

Since relaxation techniques offer benefits to a wide range of people in a wide range of clinical and non-clinical settings, with limited side effects, there is a strong research imperative to find out more about its beneficial effects and how these may be enhanced. Research is especially needed in areas such as chronic pain and insomnia, where the alternatives have tended to focus on biomedical techniques such as drugs or surgery. The ethical duty of non-maleficence (not harming) requires health professionals to use therapeutic interventions which can achieve beneficial results with the minimum of side effects. Use of relaxation techniques in clinical settings is hampered by lack of medical awareness and the emphasis, in medical training, on a biomedical model of human functioning.

Use of relaxation techniques in vulnerable populations

As well as having personal benefits, relaxation techniques can also improve moral and social development. The benefits of Vipassana meditation have been researched in drug addicts and prisoners. Were such research to be replicated, it would be important to ensure that vulnerable subjects are not coerced into participation.

Relaxation techniques can benefit children as well as adults, although the nature of these techniques requires that subjects are not cognitively impaired. Certain deep methods of relaxation should not be used on subjects suffering from serious mental disorders.

A forty-year-old man enrols for a ten-day Vipassana meditation course. He does not disclose the fact that he has been diagnosed as suffering from schizophrenia. Two days into the silent meditation he suffers from a psychotic episode during which two other students are slightly injured.

This example highlights the need to take a detailed history before using relaxation techniques. For residential courses, it may be advisable to require students to sign an undertaking that they are not suffering from a severe mental illness, or even to provide a medical certificate to that effect.

Notes

1   Vickers, A. and Zollman, C. (1999) 'ABC of Complementary Medicine. Hypnosis and Relaxation Therapies'. *British Medical Journal*. 319: 1346–1349.
2   Ibid.
3   Ibid.
4   NIH Technology Assessment Panel on Integration of Behavioural and Relaxation Approaches into the Treatment of Chronic Pain and Insomnia (1996) 'Integration of Behavioural and Relaxation Approaches into the Treatment of Chronic Pain and Insomnia'. *Journal of the Amercian Medical Association*. 276: 313–318.
5   Ibid.

24

CONCLUSION

This book has argued that CAM practitioners, as *bona fide* health care professionals, have ethical, as well as legal, duties. Analysis of the scope and content of these duties has revealed that, notwithstanding their very different therapeutic approaches, CAM practitioners work within the same ethical parameters as all other health professionals, motivated predominantly by a desire to benefit and not to cause patients harm. Whereas legal duties pose practical, though not insurmountable, challenges, most ethical responsibilities are applicable to all therapists, irrespective of the therapeutic techniques they employ. Although there may be theoretical constraints in applying western notions of morality to therapies steeped in different cultural traditions, all patients ought, nonetheless, to be able to expect that practitioners comply with basic ethical requirements.

Some therapists will no doubt argue that their forms of practice and beliefs about how to benefit patients set them apart from other health professionals and that their freedom to heal patients as they see fit should not be constrained by external regulation, whether in the form of professional codes, laws or advice on ethics. Patients, they would argue, consult them precisely because they are not doctors and because they do not work within rigid therapeutic or philosophical confines. Essentially, these practitioners wish to cling to their alternative status and maintain their separateness and otherness from conventional medicine. In the same way as they wish to remain disaffiliated from professional associations, they may resent the imposition of ethical requirements drawn from conventional bioethics and argue that they are motivated by their own personal sense of morality. These practitioners may point to high levels of patient satisfaction and the lack of complaints or litigation against CAM practitioners in support of their position. My contention is that this view is increasingly unsustainable in light of the growing trend towards integration.

Whether CAM practitioners welcome the development or not, greater integration with conventional medicine is inevitable. In some circles, the term 'integrative' or 'integrated' medicine is now replacing complementary or alternative medicine. The growing number of conventionally trained practitioners now offering CAM therapies to patients within an orthodox medical setting means that integration will proceed with or without the compliance of traditionally trained, lay practitioners. Interest in, and usage of, alternative modalities is now so significant that conventional medicine has been forced to consider how to embrace it to its advantage. Mike Saks attributes the shifts within the medical profession to their growing realisation over the last thirty years that CAM therapies could seriously impinge on the state medical monopoly on practice. He argues:

> This helps to account for the more overt attack on unorthodox medicine that developed in this period, followed by the medical incorporation of the alternatives as the elite of the profession came under growing siege from within and without in the increasingly pluralistic state political structure.[1]

Public disaffection with the medical profession, with the side effects of modern medicine and with the shortcomings of medical self-regulation, have all served to boost the popularity of CAM. Doctors are not unaware of these dissatisfactions and conventional medicine has attempted to meet these criticisms through an array of organisational changes. These include the introduction of auditing and risk management procedures, the development of more effective complaints mechanisms, improvements in accreditation, moves to enhance the public protection functions of self-regulatory bodies, and a commitment towards evidence-based practice.

At the level of the individual doctor/patient relationship, many younger practitioners embrace a more holistic approach than their predecessors and attempt to provide more patient-centred health care. An openness to the potential benefits of CAM is part of this approach. Many doctors readily accept that CAM has a role in the *overall* strategy of providing safe and effective health care. This realisation is not perceived as a threat to the dominance of conventional medicine. The edifice of modern medicine is not going to collapse merely because of the public's current enthusiasm for alternative therapies. Unsurprisingly, the approach of orthodox medicine has been to incorporate non-conventional therapies on its own terms. According to Saks:

> This is highlighted with reference to acupuncture, which has been incorporated into medicine in a selective manner as an analgesic on the basis of neurophysiological explanations, rather than as a broad-ranging practice centred on traditional Oriental philosophies.[2]

Examples of medicalised practice exist across a range of therapies. This phenomenon is in part due to the failure of CAM practitioners to conduct clinical research using methodologies consistent with CAM beliefs, leaving doctors, often in conjunction with medically qualified CAM practitioners, to conduct medicalised research which is then incorporated into conventional health care practice. Saks articulates a widespread fear amongst CAM practitioners that doctors will seek to control CAM and limit its application to the status of a medical technique within the biomedical repertoire.

The dominance of conventional medicine and the near monopoly position it enjoys with the state means that integration of alternative medicine is almost certainly likely to take the form of partial acceptance into the existing medical paradigm. The lack of cohesion between different therapies and different therapeutic organisations makes it harder for CAM to present a coherent alternative to conventional medicine and increases the risk of colonisation. CAM practitioners can still influence the form that integration may take, but they are not likely to do so by appealing to patient-preference. The spiralling costs of hi-tech, conventional medicine means that state providers are not going to accept that CAM works without evidence from research.

Moreover, in an evidence-based culture, CAM will have to demonstrate not only that their therapies work, but that they are also cost-effective. This will involve a significant shift in CAM mentality. As Stacey pointed out:

> The power of the state through legislation and policy sets the framework within which healers may practise and clients' choice be enhanced or limited. The state is interested in having a healthy population, minimally for reasons of social order. It has responsibility for the protection of clients from exploitation. *Furthermore, when the state is funding parts of the nation's health care it also has interests in the accountability of the practitioners in terms of costs as well as outcomes of treatment.*[3] (my emphasis)

Although elsewhere models of integrated health care exist in which competing belief systems flourish and are equally valued, this tends to be where the alternative modality was highly valued in the culture prior to the emergence of western, hi-tech medicine. Elsewhere, the might of modernist medicine will prevail. Integration, at least in the USA and Europe, will almost certainly take the form of conventional medicine incorporating evidence based aspects of CAM and dismissing what remains as having no place in modern, effective health care systems. This prediction is made quite explicit by Stephen E. Straus, MD, Director of the US National Institutes of Health National Center for Complementary and Alternative Medicine. His comments make disarming reading for lay CAM practitioners:

> As a result of rigorous scientific investigation, several therapeutic and preventive modalities currently deemed elements of complementary

and alternative medicine will have proven effective. Therefore, by 2020, these interventions will have been incorporated into conventional medical education and practice, and the term 'complementary and alternative medicine' will be superseded by the concept of 'integrative medicine.' ... The biological and pharmacological basis for effectiveness of selected herbal and nutritional supplements will be clarified, leading to their standardization and to the rational design of yet more potent congeners. Advances in neurobiology will elucidate mechanisms underlying ancient practices such as acupuncture and meditation, as well as the phenomenon of 'the placebo effect.' ... Other modalities will have proven unsafe or ineffective, and an informed public will have rejected them. The field of integrative medicine will be seen as providing novel insights and tools for human health, and not as a source of intellectual and philosophical tension that insinuates itself between and among practitioners of the healing arts and their patients.[4]

How alternative practitioners respond to ethics is part of a much more serious question of how they will choose to face the challenges posed by integration. Integration of CAM need not mean subordination, provided practitioners are willing to face up to fundamental problems undermining their credibility. In a culture dominated by scientific discourse, therapists who show no interest in demonstrating how their therapy works will be left behind. Dissatisfaction with existing research methodologies is not an excuse to do no research at all. CAM practitioners may be satisfied that their therapies are safe because they have been used for hundreds or even thousands of years, but this does not answer contemporary research questions of comparative efficacy, safe usage in children and compatibility with other therapeutic approaches. Whether therapies work is the central question destined to determine CAM's role in future health care. As Ernst observes:

It seems blatantly obvious that only well designed clinical investigations can establish the truth. Those who would prefer to bypass rigorous research for example, by shifting the discussion towards patients' preference and hope to integrate unproved treatments into routine health care are unlikely to succeed in the long run. Those who believe that regulation is a substitute for evidence will find that even the most meticulous regulation of nonsense must still result in nonsense. And those who insist that the evidence to support complementary and alternative medicine can legitimately be softer than in mainstream medicine will have to reconsider their position.[5]

CAM does not have to use the frameworks designed within conventional medicine, but if practitioners are dissatisfied with the models that are in

274

existence, they must design their own credible alternatives. Of course, this fundamentally depends on whether CAM practitioners wish to compete in the same area as biomedicine, namely as health care professions dedicated to promoting health and preventing disease. If CAM is content to be seen as a predominantly leisure-related, rather than health-related activity, or as a spiritual alternative to formalised religion, then few of these requirements pertain, and CAM practitioners can, for the time being, enjoy their popularity.

But to compete in the health arena requires distinct competencies which stand up to external scrutiny. Establishing that therapies work, and creating the climate and controls in which they can be practised safely by competent practitioners, is not simply a matter for ethicists, but goes to the heart of CAM's ongoing survival. If CAM practitioners want to maintain their sense of self and maintain their therapeutic integrity, they should regard the subjects discussed in this book as tools for creating a strong but separate base. Professionalisation, commitment to training and continuing professional development, research and demonstrating ethical practice are necessary ingredients to being taken seriously, which will allow CAM practitioners to compete on their own terms. The aim of this book has been to demonstrate how ethical principles can be applied in a way which is congruent with CAM practice and supportive of CAM philosophy.

Notes

1   Saks, M. (1996) 'From Quackery to Complementary Medicine: The Shifting Boundaries Between Orthodox and Unorthodox Medical Knowledge'. In Cant, S. and Sharma, U. (eds) *Complementary and Alternative Medicines. Knowledge in Practice.* Free Association Books Ltd: London.
2   Ibid.
3   Stacey, M. (1994) 'Collective Therapeutic Responsibility. Lessons From the GMC'. In Budd, S. and Sharma, U. (eds) *The Healing Bond.* Routledge: London and New York.
4   Straus, S. (1999) '2020 Vision: NIH Heads Foresee the Future'. *Journal of the American Medical Association.* 282(24), December 22/29.
5   Ernst, E. (2000) 'The Role of Complementary and Alternative Medicine'. *British Medical Journal.* 321: 1133–1135.

LIBRARY, UNIVERSITY OF CHESTER

BIBLIOGRAPHY

Bannerman, R., Burton, J. and Ch'en, W.C. (1983) *Traditional Medicine and Health Care Coverage*. World Health Organisation: Geneva.

Barton, C. and Douglas, G. (1995) *Law and Parenthood*. Butterworths: London, Dublin and Edinburgh.

Beauchamp, T.L. and Childress, J.F. (1994) *Principles of Biomedical Ethics* (4th edition). Oxford University Press: New York.

Boguslawski, M. (1979) 'The Use of Therapeutic Touch in Nursing'. *The Journal of Continuing Education in Nursing*. 10(4): 9–15.

Bowden, P. (1997) *Caring: Gender-Sensitive Ethics*. Routledge: London and New York.

British Medical Association. (2000) *Acupuncture: Efficacy, Safety and Practice*. Harwood Academic Publishers: Australia and the United Kingdom.

Budd, S. and Sharma, U. (eds) (1994) *The Healing Bond*. Routledge: London and New York.

Callender, J.S. (1998) 'Ethics and Aims in Psychotherapy: A Contribution From Kant'. *Journal of Medical Ethics*. 274.

Cant, S. and Sharma, U. (eds) (1996) *Complementary and Alternative Medicines. Knowledge in Practice*. Free Association Books Ltd: London.

Canter, D. and Nanke, L. (1991) *Psychological Aspects of Complementary Medicine. Social Aspects of Complementary Medicine*. Staffordshire: University of Keele.

Clarkson, P. (2000) *Ethics. Working with Ethical and Moral Dilemmas in Psychotherapy*. Whurr Publishers: London.

Coates, J.R. and Jobst, K.A. (eds) (1998) 'Integrated Healthcare: A Way Forward for the Next Five Years? A Discussion Document from The Prince of Wales's Initiative on Integrated Medicine'. *Journal of Alternative Complementary Medicine*. 4(2): 209–247.

Cohen, M. (1998) *Complementary and Alternative Medicine: Legal Boundaries and Regulatory Perspectives*. Johns Hopkins University Press: Baltimore, MD and London.

Dimond, B. (1998) *The Legal Aspects of Complementary Therapy Practice*. Churchill Livingstone: Edinburgh.

Egan, E.C. (1998) 'Therapeutic Touch'. In Snyder, M. and Lindquist, R. (eds) *Complementary and Alternative Therapies in Nursing* (3rd edition). Springer Publishing Company Inc.: New York.

276

Eisenberg, D., Kessler, R.C. and Foster, C. (1993) 'Unconventional Medicine in the United States'. *New England Journal of Medicine*. 328: 246–252.

Eisenberg, D., with Wright, T.L. (1995) *Encounters with Qi. Exploring Chinese Medicine*. W.W. Norton & Co, Inc.: New York.

Eisenberg, D.M., Davis, R.B. and Ettner, S.I., *et al.* (1998) 'Trends in Alternative Medicine Use in the United States, 1990–1997: Results of a Follow-up National Survey'. *Journal of the American Medical Association*. 280: 1569–1575.

Featherstone, C. and Forsyth, L. (1997) *Medical Marriage: The New Partnership Between Orthodox and Complementary Medicine*. Findhorn Press: Findhorn, Scotland.

Gillon, R. (1986) *Philosophical Medical Ethics*. John Wiley & Sons: Chichester.

Glover, J. (2000) *Humanity. A Moral History of the Twentieth Century*. Yale University Press: New Haven, CT.

Greenhalgh, T. and Hurwitz, B. (1998) *Narrative Based Medicine: Dialogue and Discourse in Clinical Practice*. BMJ Publishing: London.

Hawkins, P. and Shohet, R. (eds) (1989) *Supervision in the Helping Professions*. Open University Press: Milton Keynes.

Holmes, J. and Lindley, R. (1998) *The Values of Psychotherapy* (revised edition). Karnac Books: London.

House of Lords. Sixth Report of the House of Lords Science and Technology Committee. (2000) *Complementary and Alternative Medicine*. London: The Stationery Office.

Humber, J. and Almeder, R. (eds) (1988) *Alternative Medicine and Ethics*. Humana Press: Totowa, NJ.

James, K. (1988) 'Aromatherapy'. In Snyder, M. and Lindquist, R. (eds) *Complementary Alternative Therapies in Nursing* (3rd edition). Springer Publishing Company Inc.: New York

Jehu, D. (1994) *Patients as Victims, Sexual Abuse in Psychotherapy and Counselling*. John Wiley & Sons: Chichester and New York.

Jenkins, P. (1997) *Counselling, Psychotherapy and the Law*. Sage: London.

Johannessen, H. (1996) 'Individualized Knowledge: Reflexologists, Biopaths and Kinesiologists in Denmark'. In Cant, S and Sharma, U (eds) *Complementary and Alternative Medicines. Knowledge in Practice*. Free Association Books Ltd: London.

Koehn, D. (1994) *The Ground of Professional Ethics*. Routledge: London and New York.

Kolb, D.A., Rubin, I.M. and McIntyre, J.M. (1971) *Organizational Psychology: An Experiential Approach*. Prentice Hall: New York.

Kolb, D. (1984) *Experiential Learning*. Prentice Hall: New York.

Kuhn, T.S. (1970) *The Structure of Scientific Revolutions*. University of Chicago Press, Chicago, IL.

Lewith, G.T. and Aldridge, D. (eds) (1993) *Clinical Research Methodology for Complementary Therapies*. Hodder and Stoughton: Sevenoaks.

Martindale, B., Morner, M., Rodriguez, M. and Vidit, J. (eds) (1997) *Supervision and Its Vicissitudes*. Karnac Books: London.

Micozzi, M. (ed.) (1996) *Fundamentals of Complementary and Alternative Medicine*. Churchill Livingstone: Edinburgh.

Mojay, G. (1996) *Aromatherapy for Healing the Spirit*. Gaia Books Ltd: Stroud.

Morgan, D., Glanville, H., Mars, S. and, Nathanson, V. (1988) 'Education and Training in Complementary and Alternative Medicine: A Postal Survey of UK Universities, Medical Schools and Faculties of Nurse Education'. *Complementary Therapeutic Medicine*. 6: 64–70.

Nelson, H.L. (1997) *Stories and their Limits. Narrative Approaches to Bioethics*. Routledge: London and New York.

Nessa, J. and Malterud, K. (1988) 'Tell Me What's Wrong With Me: A Discourse Analysis Approach to the Concept of Patient Autonomy'. *Journal of Medical Ethics*. 24: 394–400.

Newell, C.A., Anderson, L.A. and Phillipson, J.D. (1996) *Herbal Medicines. A Guide for Health Care Professionals*. The Pharmaceutical Press: London.

Pantanowitz, D. (1994) *Alternative Medicine. A Doctor's Perspective*. Southern Book Publishers, South Africa.

Pope, K.S. (1998) 'How Clients are Harmed by Sexual Contact with Mental Health Professionals: The Syndrome and its Prevalence'. *Journal of Counselling and Development*. 67: 222–226.

Pope, K.S., Sonne, J.L. and Holroyd, J. (1993) *Sexual Feelings in Psychotherapy: Explorations for Therapists and Therapists-in-training*. American Psychological Association: Washington, DC.

Pope, K.S. and Vasquez, M. (1998) *Ethics in Psychotherapy and Counseling. A Practical Guide* (2nd edition). Jossey-Bass: San Francisco, CA.

Purtilo, R. (1999) *Ethical Dimensions in the Health Professions* (3rd edition). W.B. Saunders & Co.: London.

Rankin-Box, D. (1995) *The Nurses' Handbook of Complementary Therapies*. Churchill Livingstone: Edinburgh.

Rippere, V. and Williams, R. (1985) *Wounded Healers – Mental Health Workers' Experiences of Depression*. John Wiley & Sons: Chichester.

Saks, M. (1995) *Professions and the Public Interest. Medical Power, Altruism and Alternative Medicine*. Routledge: London and New York

Savalescu, J. and Momeyer, R.W. (1997) 'Should Informed Consent Be Based On Rational Beliefs?'. *Journal of Medical Ethics*. 23(5): 282–288.

Schoener, G. (1998) 'Assessment and Rehabilitation of Professionals Who Violate Sexual Boundaries With Clients'. In *Collected Papers on Professional Misconduct*. In Good Faith & Associates: North Melbourne, Victoria, Australia.

Schön, D. (1983) *The Reflective Practitioner. How Professionals Think in Action*. Avebury: Aldershot.

Schwartz, R. (1995) 'Life Style, Health Status, and Distributive Justice'. In Grubb, A. and Mehlman, M. (eds) *Justice and Health Care: Comparative Perspectives*. John Wiley & Sons: Chichester and New York.

Sharma, U. (1992) *Complementary Medicine Today: Practitioners and Patients*. Tavistock, Routledge: London and New York.

Sheldon, S. and Thomson, M. (1998) *Feminist Perspectives on Health Care Law*. Cavendish: London and Sydney.

Singer, P. (ed.) (1991) *A Companion to Ethics*. Blackwell: Oxford.

Snyder, M. and Lindquist, R. (eds) (1998) *Complementary Alternative Therapies in Nursing* (3rd edition). Springer Publishing Company Inc.: New York

Spencer, J.W. and Jacobs, J.J. (1999) *Complementary/Alternative Medicine. An Evidence-Based Approach*. Mosby: St Louis, MO.

Stevensen, C. (1995) 'Aromatherapy'. In. Rankin-Box, D. (ed.) *The Nurses' Handbook of Complementary Therapies*. Churchill Livingstone: Edinburgh: 51–58.

Stone, J. and Matthews, J. (1996) *Complementary Medicine and the Law*. Oxford University Press: New York.

Thomas, K.J., Carr, J., Westlake, L. and Williams, B.T. (1991) 'Use of Non-orthodox and Conventional Health Care in Great Britain'. *British Medical Journal*. 302 (6770): 2007–2010.

Thomas, K.J., Fall, M. and Nicholl J. (1995) 'National Survey of Access to Complementary Therapies via General Practice'. Report to Department of Health. Medical Care Research Unit, SCHARR, Regent Court, 30 Regent Street, Sheffield, SI 4DA.

Tisserand, R. and Balacs, T. (1995) *Essential Oil Safety: A Guide for Health Care Professionals*. Churchill Livingstone: Edinburgh.

United Kingdom Central Council for Nursing, Midwifery and Health Visiting (1996) *Guidelines for Professional Practice*. UKCC: London.

Vickers, A. (1996) *Massage and Aromatherapy: A Guide for Health Professionals*. Chapman Hall: London.

Vincent, C. and Furnham, A. (1997) *Complementary Medicine. A Research Perspective*. John Wiley & Sons: Chichester.

INDEX

280